The Feminine Touch

THOMAS A. QUINN

The Feminine Touch
Women in Osteopathic Medicine

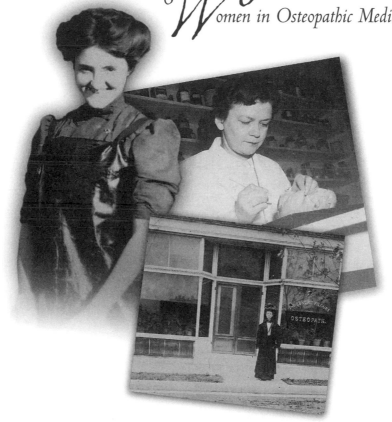

Truman State University Press

Cover: All images from Museum of Osteopathic Medicine (SM), clockwise from top left: dissection class, ca. 1908 [2000.34.03 ca 1908]; female osteopathic student in a dissection class, ca. 1912 [PH292]; Lenora Kilgore, DO in front of her office, ca. 1910 [2002.06.01]; Eva Manning and Lorraine Peissner, Jan.1975 [2010.02.895]; Olwen Gutensohn, DO [2020.02.846].

Title page: All images from Museum of Osteopathic Medicine (SM), clockwise from top left: female osteopathic student in a dissection class, ca. 1912 [PH292]; Olwen Gutensohn, DO [2020.02.846]; Lenora Kilgore, DO in front of her office, ca. 1910 [2002.06.01].

Unless otherwise noted, portraits were provided by the person depicted. All reasonable attempts have been made to contact the copyright holders of historical images. If you believe you are the copyright holder, please contact Truman State University Press.

Cover design: Teresa Wheeler

Library of Congress Cataloging-in-Publication Data

Quinn, Thomas A., 1940–
The feminine touch : women in osteopathic medicine / Thomas A. Quinn.
    p. ; cm.
Includes bibliographical references and index.
ISBN 978-1-935503-13-2 (pbk. : alk. paper) ISBN 978-1-612480-26-8 (ebook)
1. Osteopathic medicine—History. 2. Women in medicine—History—19th century. 3. Women in medicine—History—20th century. 4. Women in medicine—History—21st century. I. Title.
[DNLM: 1. Osteopathic Medicine—history. 2. History, 19th Century. 3. History, 20th Century. 4. History, 21st Century. 5. Osteopathic Physicians—history. 6. Women—history. WB 112]
RZ321.Q85 2011
615.5'33—dc23

                                                                                    2011015107

The Touch

EVERYONE CAN TOUCH BUT NOT EVERYONE has "The Touch." In the early stages of learning to perform osteopathic manipulative medicine, the student must first be taught the art of palpation, the ability to touch and to know what you are feeling. It is easy to touch, but it takes months or even years to be able to discriminate fine differences in tissue changes. But to imply that "The Touch" consists only of the ability to palpate and to distinguish fine changes in tissue is to tell only half of the story. Touch is a two-way system. Palpation is the ability to detect information from the patient's body by way of the physician's hands, which tell her or him about changes that have taken place within the patient's body. A person who has The Touch has the ability to heal with their hands. The *healing touch*, the *gentle touch*, the *therapeutic touch*, the *human touch* are just some of the terms used to describe the phenomenon of healing with the hands.

Explanations for this phenomenon vary widely. Some attribute a metaphysical or magical quantity to The Touch, others ascribe a religious connection, and yet others offer a psychosomatic explanation. In the nineteenth century, there were those who referred to themselves as magnetic healers, implying that they healed patients using magnetism or some force that passed through their hands to the patient. There is much we do not understand and much that continues to defy scientific explanation; although there is not yet any scientific explanation for "The Touch," it is difficult to deny that such a thing exists.

Dr. A. T. Still lived and worked during the era of magnetic healers, mesmerists, spiritualists, and bonesetters. He was influenced by alternative medical practices, but ultimately he rejected them along with the mainstream medical treatments of his day, and developed a distinctive form of medical practice that has matured into modern, scientific osteopathic medicine. Dr. Still believed that women had a special quality, a gentleness of touch, which he recognized as "The Feminine Touch," that made women natural healers. For this reason, he opened wide the doors of osteopathy to women. Blanche Still, his youngest daughter, wrote,

> There is no science more beautiful than osteopathy, none better adapted to women whose delicate sense of touch makes her qualified for its study and practice.

Contents

Foreword

WHEN I FIRST MET DR. QUINN as he embarked on the research for this book at the Still National Osteopathic Museum, his love of osteopathy and its history was immediately evident—and infectious. Spending several summer months here in Kirksville with his wife, Sissy, Dr. Quinn pored through virtually everything in our collection regarding women in this profession. In the process, his work has greatly enhanced our own understanding of that remarkable history—a history that is indeed alive and ever-expanding as we continue to learn more about the extraordinary women who blazed the trail for today's more than 29 percent* female practitioners in the United States.

Here at the museum we are frequently asked, "Were women always in osteopathy?" And the answer, of course, is "YES!" Beginning in 1892 with the original six pioneering females who enrolled in the school's first class (which included one of founder A. T. Still's own daughters, Martha Helen "Blanche" Still) women have continued to constitute a major force in the successful growth of the osteopathic profession. Even though Blanche Still never established a practice because of her eventual roles as both the wife of Dr. George M. Laughlin (surgeon and later president of the school) and as primary caregiver for her aging parents, Blanche eventually blazed her own distinct trails as editor of the *Journal of Osteopathy*, as well as a trustee and assistant secretary of the American School of Osteopathy (now A. T. Still University). In 1898 she wrote:

> "Will it injure a lady's social standing to study Osteopathy?" [This] question was asked not long ago by a lady of refinement and education... To answer the question we will ask another: "Does intelligence in this day and age injure a lady's social standing?"
>
> ...Society is no longer a mere gathering of butterflies to flirt and gossip; society today demands brains. The diamonds of a wealthy woman may shine brightly, but if she has no intelligence they will

---

* AOA, Osteopathic Medical Profession Report, June 2008

soon lose their luster. Osteopathy is the brightest gem in the diadem of intelligence that crowns the queen of society…

No, a thousand times no; Osteopathy does not injure a lady's social standing among people who have intelligence enough to belong to good society. Osteopathy is elevating, lady-like, noble and true, and instead of an injury provides a means of advancement. Ladies should have no fears that the study will injure them socially, morally, or financially.

Hailing osteopathy as a way for women to utilize their intellect as well as their natural nurturing tendencies, Dr. Still wrote:

I have always felt a determination to hunt until I could find a suitable position which I could recommend to our women. I believe I have made the discovery…. [M]an has within him all the qualities for ease and comfort, and when disease makes them uncomfortable, he or she who is familiar with the machinery of life can give them ease and comfort and restore the person to good health. In the case of the ladies, they have proven their ability to adjust the human body. She gets her pay and is proud of her diploma, proud of her being and proud of her position…

—*Journal of Osteopathy*, December 1898

In this book, Dr. Quinn examines the careers of early American School of Osteopathy women graduates who rose to prominence in the osteopathic field, including Jeanette "Nettie" Hubbard Bolles, founder of the Bolles Institute of Osteopathy in 1897; Louisa Burns, renowned osteopathic medical researcher; Josephine Peirce, founder of the Osteopathic Women's National Association; and Florence McCoy, the first osteopath to give expert testimony in a court of law. By looking at womens' contributions to the critical early days of osteopathy, Dr. Quinn uncovers how the traditionally male-dominated profession of medicine opened up to women and how "those women" took the reins of Still's new discovery, raising osteopathy to the highest levels in the medical world today.

Debra Loguda Summers, Curator
Museum of Osteopathic Medicine (SM)

Preface and Acknowledgments

Whenever my siblings or I fell ill, my mother, like any good parent, dutifully and anxiously took us to the doctor's office. That type of trip is a childhood memory everyone seems to share without significant variation, from the starched white physician's frock to the stainless steel instruments gleaming from the counter with cold and sterile indifference. One particular visit, however, was different, and my mother had an unusual reason to be anxious that day. It was the closing days of World War II and many MDs had been called into service for the war effort, so there were painfully few physicians available for the home front. I was only four at the time, but my mother tells me that I had a high fever and she was especially anxious because this physician was an osteopath, and she was afraid he would send us home with some strange potion or incantation. To her great relief, the osteopath examined me and prescribed the very same medication our regular pediatrician did.

That single visit summed up my entire life experience with osteopathic medicine until I was a college undergraduate applying to medical schools in my hometown of Philadelphia. One by one, I visited each of the medical schools in the Philadelphia area (with the exception of the Women's Medical College, which at the time did not accept male students). One day, I visited the Philadelphia College of Osteopathy (PCO) on 48th and Spruce Streets on the way to my evening job as a clerk in the emergency department of a local hospital, which I needed to help pay my tuition at LaSalle College (now LaSalle University). There I met Marguerite Archer, the assistant registrar, who greeted me warmly and took her time to answer all of my questions, which were numerous. She took me on a tour of the medical college and showed me the hospital that was attached to the college. She then introduced me to the registrar, Tom Rowland. That evening the emergency room was unusually quiet and so, not having any excuse not to, I opened the information I had picked up at the osteopathic college. The chief resident of the hospital, with whom I was well acquainted from our days as Boy Scout camp counselors, happened into the room at that moment and saw the literature. To say that he became upset would be a gross understatement. For the next several months, every time I was working, he would find a reason to come to the emergency department to try to convince me that I would be committing an egregious error if I enrolled in an osteopathic medical school.

PCO was located between LaSalle College and the hospital where I worked. Since I had to pass the school on my way to work, it was a simple matter for me to stop in the osteopathic college's library to seek answers to the many questions and arguments my friend raised with the sincere intent of protecting me from making what he considered to be the worst mistake of my life. The librarian and I were soon on a first-name basis.

The following year, in September 1962, I found myself a member of the freshman class of PCO. The decision to enroll in PCO would prove momentous for me in many ways, this book being just one outcome of my choosing a career in osteopathic medicine. Now it happens that there was only one female student in my medical school class. At the time, I didn't think much of the fact that this would be the first time I had ever attended a class with a woman. I had been educated in parochial schools and at the time I attended LaSalle College, it was still an all-male college. So it was only while doing research for this book that I learned that 1966, the year I graduated from medical school, was the low point for female enrollment in American medical schools in the twentieth century.[1]

During my senior year at PCO, I had my first opportunity to sift through the unique history of the profession, writing "The History of the Philadelphia College of Osteopathy" for my senior yearbook, *Synapses* 1966. My interest in research led me years later to serve as faculty advisor for the Student Osteopathic Research Association at the Lake Erie College of Osteopathic Medicine, Bradenton (LECOM Bradenton), where I encouraged students to study the history of their profession. In 2006, I organized a month-long research trip to the Still National Osteopathic Museum (since renamed the Museum of Osteopathic Medicine) and the International Center for Osteopathic History, both located at A. T. Still University, Kirksville College of Osteopathic Medicine, in Kirksville, Missouri. That school is the modern successor to the first osteopathic medical school founded by Andrew Taylor Still in 1892.

My initial plan was to take four medical students and my wife with me. We applied for research grants to defray expenses for the medical students, but when we failed to secure funding, all but one of the students dropped out. In the end, my wife, Sissy, and April Smith-Gonzalez, who had just completed her first year at LECOM Bradenton, traveled with me to the birthplace of osteopathy. We spent the next month deep in the collection of the museum and the International Center for

1 Duffy, *The Healers*, 36.

Osteopathic History, where the museum staff, most notably curator Debra Loguda-Summers and executive director Jason Haxton, graciously assisted with our research. Without their help and the vast stores of information available in the archives of the museum, this book would not have been possible.

I had originally planned to write a series of articles about the history of the profession, as material on the subject was sorely lacking. I also thought of compiling a definitive pictorial history of the profession; however several pictorial publications had already been done, and though a more complete book would be a worthwhile project, it would have been duplication. Fortunately, both Sissy and April encouraged me to look into the history of women in the profession, perhaps inspired by the multitude of historic pictures in the hallways that bore testament to the acceptance of women students from the very first class. It was impressive to see not only the early and consistent enrollment of women students, but also the high number of female students enrolled through the history of the school. I learned that the most complete work on women in osteopathic medicine was a thirty-two page pamphlet written by Georgia Walter in 1991, and though numerous journal articles had also been published, there was no complete study of the role of women in osteopathy. I had found a gap in the historical dialogue: the reciprocal role of women and the osteopathic profession. Sissy suggested the title "The Feminine Touch." Thus I started on a five-year journey that has resulted in the publication of this book.

There have been many more female osteopathic physicians who have made significant contributions throughout the decades than could possibly be included in this work. I intend no slight to their contributions. Some women have been omitted because their stories are told elsewhere; some modern women were omitted because I was unable to obtain sufficient information from them. Most of the women in this book have contributed positively to the advancement of osteopathic medicine. There were a few women who contributed negatively, and if that contribution was significant, I included them. Most notable among these was the notorious Dr. Zeo Wilkins, the most disreputable and infamous DO to ever exist (see chapter 3).

I contacted every specialty college of osteopathic medicine in an attempt to acquire a representative sample of significant female DOs in each specialty. Some colleges and specialty organizations suggested candidates for the book and some ignored the request. My most important sources, however, were female physicians who recommended other women who had made significant contributions to the profession; I wish to thank everyone who submitted names for consideration. I also wish to thank Gary Laco, PhD, who proofread the manuscript, and Matthew Nelson, a LECOM Bradenton medical student who provided original research into the osteopathic-chiropractic connections. Most importantly, I wish to thank Jeffery Wang, a LECOM Bradenton medical student, who assisted in putting together the final draft of the book.

There are several terms that are used throughout this book that may not be familiar to persons not knowledgeable in medical history. For this reason I have included a glossary of terms.

Chapter One

Women and Medical Education

"Surely this is a little difficult. We are told that the great objection to women entering professional life was that they would not care to marry, hence the desire to keep them out. Now conditions are reversed and the objection is that they do. Really, it is not easy to please."

The 1893 Women's Medical Journal

"In sickness there is nothing so soothing as the gentle touch of a woman's hand. Then why not train her hand that she may do her work intelligently and scientifically?"

Mary Conner, DO

OSTEOPATHY WAS BORN INTO THE WORLD at a time when the professional practice of medicine was the dominion of privileged males who controlled every aspect of the profession. According to the intellectual reasoning of the time, science was masculine by its very nature and was therefore not an appropriate domain for women, who with few exceptions were excluded from pursuing careers in science and medicine.

The participation of women in science and medicine has a long and complex history, complicated by Western ideas of femininity and the appropriate role of women, and women's access to education. In the Middle Ages, convents offered women an opportunity to pursue their education, including the study of medicine, but their talents usually remained within the walls of their convent. From their origins in the twelfth century, European universities, on the other hand, were closed to women. The universities were established to train men to enter careers in government, law, teaching, medicine, or the church, and women were not expected to enter these professions. There were rare exceptions—usually women who studied and worked with a father or husband—but most women simply did not have access to advanced learning. For men, physical strength was valued more highly than intellectual prowess, and women were expected to focus on household management and domestic affairs. It was not until the sixteenth century that education for its own sake was seen as an appropriate pursuit for the leisured classes. When royal courts and aristocratic households began to sponsor artists, poets, philosophers, and inventors, learning moved to a domestic environment, with men engaging in government and martial activities and women engaging in intellectual pursuits. Despite their increased involvement in learning, it was still rare for a woman to pursue an education in a public setting or to pursue a career outside of her family circle. Women who pursued intellectual activities often focused on the arts, as subjects such as science and mathematics were seen as unfeminine.

Various reasons were given to explain why science was considered an inappropriate pursuit for women. In her study of women in science, Londa Schiebinger explains, "In the seventeenth century, English natural philosopher Margaret Cavendish spoke for many when she wrote that women's minds were simply too 'cold' and 'soft' to sustain rigorous thought…. In the late eighteenth century, the female cranial cavity was supposed to be too small to hold powerful brains; in the late nineteenth century, the exercise of women's brains was said to shrivel their ovaries."[1] On the other hand, American physician Benjamin Rush, in his 1787 *Thoughts upon Female Education*, argued that a woman should be educated so that she would be "an agreeable companion for a sensible man" and would ensure her husband's "perseverance in the paths of rectitude," and called for loyal "republican mothers" to instruct "their sons in the principles of liberty and government." For Rush, the issue was not whether women were capable of intellectual pursuits, but to what use they should put their education.

Early Female Physicians in Europe

In 1754, Dorothea Erxleben became the first woman to receive a medical degree from a European university. Her father, a medical doctor, had encouraged her studies throughout her childhood. She studied medicine with her father and with her brother as he prepared for university. When her brother entered the university, Dorothea petitioned Fredrick II of Prussia for special permission to accompany him, a petition that was granted in April 1741. In response to this auspicious event, a pamphlet was circulated to protest a woman entering the medical profession, asserting that women were forbidden by law to practice medicine and, therefore, should not receive a university

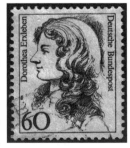

Stamp commemorating Dorothea Erxleben, issued in 1987 as part of the Women in German History series.

degree. Dorothea responded in kind in 1742 by publishing *Inquiry into the Causes Preventing the Female Sex from Studying*. Others offered a form of support, recommending that a separate university be founded for women or that women be taught in separate classrooms. Unfortunately, the outbreak of war prevented Dorothea from attending university at that time, but she continued to study and in 1754 she passed her doctoral exam and received her license to practice medicine. It was nearly a century and a half before another woman would graduate from the University of Halle's School of Medicine.[2]

In 1812, a young medical student named James Miranda Stewart (or Stuart) Barry presented his doctoral dissertation on femoral hernias to the University of Edinburgh and was awarded a degree in medicine. In reality, this medical student was a young woman (probably Margaret Ann Bulkley, a niece of artist James Barry), who was in her early teens when she entered the university in 1809. She spent the remainder of her life disguised as a male and had a successful career as a British military surgeon, where she was known as a skillful physician, a brilliant surgeon, and an advocate of medical reform. Barry served

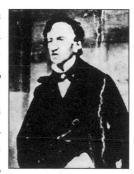

James Barry, MD

first in South Africa, where she performed the first successful Cesarean section in the British Empire. Barry eventually rose to the rank of inspector general of the Army Medical Department, serving as chief medical doctor in Canada at the end of a career that spanned four decades.

Biographers speculate that some may have suspected or even known Barry's true gender, but most simply considered the doctor very eccentric and somewhat effeminate. Barry was also known to be quarrelsome and fought at least one duel over a matter of honor. While serving in the Crimea, Barry had an encounter with Florence Nightingale, who described Dr. Barry as behaving "like a brute." Dr. Barry hid her gender so successfully that her secret was not made public until after her death in 1865. The woman who prepared the body for the funeral ignored Barry's request that she not be changed out of the clothing she was wearing when she died, and reported her discovery that Barry was not only completely female, but also had borne a child. The story was reported in the press, but Barry was interred without a postmortem, so it was impossible to verify. The medical community eventually decided that Barry must have been a male hermaphrodite. Apparently it was impossible for them to believe a woman could have been a good doctor.[3]

MEDICINE IN THE NEW WORLD

While upper-class Europeans were relying on professional physicians, surgeons, and apothecaries, those less privileged often relied on folk remedies and self-care. In colonial America, women traditionally assumed the roles of caregiver and healer within their homes and their communities, nurturing the young, the old, and the invalid. There were also professional physicians; however, before universities, professional societies, and licensing agencies were established, anybody could call himself a doctor and set up a practice. Some aspiring physicians traveled to Europe for training, then returned to the colonies to practice, and some physicians studied medicine through an apprenticeship with an established physician. Still others trained as physicians in Europe and chose to settle and set up a practice in the New World, but university-trained physicians were generally middle- or upper-class and few were willing to leave lucrative careers in Europe for an uncertain future in the New World.

The first college in the New World, Harvard College, was founded in 1636 to train Puritan ministers. By the mid-eighteenth century, various religious denominations had established colleges to train ministers for their churches. While most university-educated men had gained at least some medical knowledge, it was not until the mid-eighteenth century that the colonies were established enough that colleges and universities could be founded that focused specifically on medical training.

The first medical school in the New World was established at the College of Philadelphia in 1765. This school, which would later become the prestigious University of Pennsylvania School of Medicine, brought the European tradition of male exclusivity to the medical profession of America. By the time of the American Revolution, there were many local medical societies that promoted the professionalization of medicine and several colonies had laws for licensing medical practitioners.

By 1800, there were about a dozen schools in the United States that granted medical degrees and the practice of medicine had been largely taken over by men, being seen as a profession requiring scientific expertise and formal training—something only available to the more elite segments of society. Physicians who had studied at a college or university and apprenticed with an established physician saw themselves as skilled professionals, forming medical societies and advocating medical licensing to protect their position in society. On the frontiers, however, such physicians were in short supply, and many practitioners had trained only through apprenticeships or self-study. This also meant that some women were able to practice medicine despite the opposition of professional gentleman physicians.

The increasing professionalization of medicine also meant that physicians replaced midwives for obstetrical care. This is especially ironic given that ideas of feminine modesty meant that male physicians could not visually examine women with gynecological problems; when delivering a baby they would drape the woman with a sheet, assisting in the delivery only by placing their hands under this partition.

In the 1820s, Samuel Thomson, an herbalist, traveled throughout New Hampshire, treating poorer families who could not afford the high prices of a doctor. His herbal concoctions began to gain a reputation as effective treatments, and soon families from distant towns began to travel to him to acquire his elixirs. This form of medical practice became known as Thomsonian Medicine and was based on Thomson's rejection of the medical community's practices, which he considered to be exclusionary. Alternative medicines gained in popularity as part of the wave of egalitarian antielitism that dominated the 1830s. Leaders of what became known as the popular health movement argued that even the lenient standards of licensing medical practitioners in the nineteenth century were too restrictive for the new ideals of personal freedom in the new American republic, declaring that "In a free country, anyone should have the right to practice medicine." As a result of this movement, by 1845 there were only three states that had laws regulating the practice of medicine,[4] and the licensing of medical physicians in the United States became practically nonexistent. Because apprenticeship was a common and widely accepted method of receiving a medical education, many medical practitioners had never attended medical school. For the next several decades, it became possible for practically any individual to practice medicine, almost anywhere in the United States[5]—as long as they were male.

As the formal practice of medicine became more scientific and professionalized, other types of medicine proliferated: herbalism, bonesetting, folk medicine, self-care, Thompsonian medicine, homeopathy, hydropathy, physiomedicalism, and eclectic medicine, as well as the usual array of techniques practiced by quacks and charlatans. Of the practitioners of these different approaches, the homeopaths, eclectics, and physiomedicals all granted the MD degree to their students. The orthodox physicians who also used the MD degree referred to themselves as "regular physicians" or "the regulars," and referred to other MD groups as "irregular physicians" or "the irregulars." The founder of homeopathic medicine, Samuel Hahnemann, referred to orthodox physicians as "allopathic physicians" or "allopaths," a name that has remained and is used to identify MD physicians of today.

The new forms of medicine reflected the growing antielitist movement; and as part of it, the popular health movement encouraged ordinary people to take control of their own health care and rejected the notion of licensing of medical practitioners. At the same time, medicine itself was undergoing tremendous changes, with knowledge gleaned from the study of anatomy, physiology, and pathology leading to new treatments that gradually replaced the older practices of bleeding, blistering, purging, vomiting, and sweating to eliminate bad humors and restore humoral balance. Throughout all of these changes in the practice of medicine, the strength and talent of a few exceptional women and the support of a few forward-thinking men began to crack the barriers preventing women from taking their rightful place in the professional practice of medicine. One of the unsung champions of women's equality was Dr. Andrew Taylor Still, whose new osteopathic profession created opportunities for American women to practice medicine equally alongside their male colleagues.[6]

First Female Physicians in America

According to *Daughters of America; or, Women of the Century,* published in 1882, "Among the first, if not the first, to practise medicine in this country, was Dr. Harriot K. Hunt."[7] Hunt's story illustrates the double standard applied to women in medicine. Hunt received her medical education through an apprenticeship and set up a practice with her sister in Boston in 1835, fourteen years before Elizabeth Blackwell became the first female in America to receive a medical degree. In her autobiography, Hunt notes, "In October, 1835, we removed to the corner of Spring and Leverett streets, where we lived some time, advertised, and began, as it were, our profession."[8] Because she was a

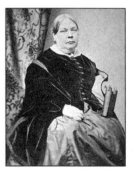

Harriot Kezia Hunt, MD (Hon.)
[Schlesinger Library, Radcliffe Institute, Harvard University]

woman, however, her male peers never acknowledged her as a physician, despite the fact that approximately 75 percent of male physicians of the time had themselves never attended medical school.[9]

In 1847, Harriot Hunt was denied admission to Harvard Medical School. She applied again in 1850 and was initially admitted, but was forced to withdraw due to protests from male students who drew a resolution stating:

> Resolved that no woman of true delicacy would be willing, in the presence of men, to listen to the discussion of subjects necessary to come under medicine.

RESOLVED that we are not opposed to allowing woman her rights, but do protest against her appearing in places where her presence is calculated to destroy our respect for the modesty and delicacy of her sex.[10]

Another ninety-five years would pass before a woman would finally be accepted into Harvard Medical School in 1945. In recognition of her longstanding medical practice, in 1853 the Female Medical College of Pennsylvania awarded Harriot Hunt an honorary medical degree.[11]

The first woman to receive a formal degree in medicine in the United States was Elizabeth Blackwell, who earned an MD degree in 1849.[12] This was a great achievement during an era when women were expected to behave modestly, and the subjects of anatomy and physiology were considered inappropriate for women, who were thought to be modest and pure by nature. The restrictive social atmosphere, together with lax legal requirements allowing any man to call himself a physician, resulted in an overcrowded and male-dominated medical profession.[13] At the same time, some were calling for changes in the status of women. In 1787, founding father Benjamin Rush wrote

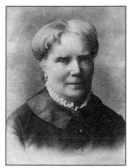

Elizabeth Blackwell, MD, undated portrait [Hobart and William Smith Colleges Archives]

a tract endorsing education for women, although he did not think women should pursue careers. And in England, Mary Wollstonecraft published *A Vindication of the Rights of Woman* in 1792. In the early 1800s, schools for women began to spring up around the country, and by the 1820s, women were entering the teaching profession. The women's movement grew alongside the temperance and abolition movements, holding its first national convention in Seneca Falls, New York, in 1848, one year before the first woman graduated from an American medical school.

It was during this time of conflicting social attitudes about gender that the eleven-year-old Elizabeth Blackwell came to America from England with her family. Her forward-thinking father made sure that she and her sisters received the same education as their brothers. Blackwell taught school for several years, but a friend who was dying of cancer encouraged her to study medicine, asserting that a woman physician would have given her more comfort than her male doctor. Elizabeth studied with physicians in South Carolina and Philadelphia while looking for a medical school that would admit her, in part because as a woman she could not gain recognition as a physician even after completing her apprenticeship. Blackwell reasoned that if, in conjunction with her apprenticeship, she graduated from a medical school with a formal medical education, then she would gain recognition as a legitimate physician.[14]

After being turned down by multiple medical schools, Blackwell applied to the Geneva Medical School of Western New York in 1847. When the administration received her application, they were perplexed. Unsure of how to proceed, they decided to put her application to the vote of the medical students. The notion of a woman attending medical school was so unthinkable that the students believed the school administration was playing a prank on them, and so they unintentionally voted to accept her. When the students discovered that this was a genuine application, they were dismayed and outraged, but it was too late. By voting to accept Elizabeth Blackwell into the medical school, they left an unintended mark upon American medical history.[15]

Overcoming the barrage of resentment and scorn from her professors and fellow students, Elizabeth Blackwell successfully graduated in 1849, becoming the first woman in America to receive a medical degree. Once Dr. Blackwell had led the way, other medical schools, especially those associated with alternative medicines, began to accept female students. But receiving a medical degree did not guarantee that a woman could establish a practice and be accepted by her fellow doctors. Following graduation, in spite of having graduated first in her class, Dr. Blackwell could not find any hospital that would admit her for clinical training and was forced to return to England. In 1851, Dr. Blackwell returned to New York to start her practice, but was denied privileges at every hospital where she applied. In addition, landlords refused to rent her an office, wishing to avoid the stigma of renting to a female physician. Not to be deterred, Dr. Blackwell purchased a house in a slum area of New York City and opened the New York Infirmary for the Treatment of Women and Children. Her younger sister Emily, along with Marie Zakrzewska, both recent graduates of Cleveland Medical College, soon joined her practice and the infirmary flourished.[16]

In 1849, the same year that Dr. Blackwell graduated, Sarah Adamson applied to the Geneva Medical School of Western New York in an attempt to follow Blackwell's precedent. Again, the faculty put the application to a student vote. This time, alas, the students had grown weary of their unintended claim to fame and immediately rejected the application. Until it closed in 1871, the Geneva Medical School of Western New York never admitted another woman.[17] The Central Medical College of New York, an eclectic medical school in Syracuse, did, however, admit three women in 1849 and Sarah Adamson become the third woman in America to earn her medical degree in 1851 and the first to complete a hospital internship in 1852.[18]

In 1864, Rebecca Davis Lee Crumpler became the first black female physician when she graduated from the New England Female Medical College. Crumpler left few records behind, and for many years scholars designated Rebecca Cole, who received her degree from the Woman's Medical College of Pennsylvania in 1867, the first black female physician. In the first medical book published by a black American, Crumpler described her early career and education:

> Having been reared by a kind aunt in Pennsylvania, whose usefulness with the sick was continually sought, I early conceived a liking for, and sought every opportunity to be in a position to relieve the sufferings of others. Later in life I devoted my time, when best I could, to nursing as a business, serving under different doctors for a period of eight years (from '52 to '60); most of the time at my adopted home in Charlestown, Middlesex County, Massachusetts. From these doctors I received letters commending me to the faculty of the New England Female Medical College, whence, four years afterward, I received the degree of Doctress of Medicine.

The first black medical school did not open until 1868, and until that time, medical schools typically denied admission to black applicants, so the support of her employers clearly played an important role in her ability to enter medical school. After the end of the American Civil War in 1865, Dr. Crumpler moved to Richmond, Virginia, where she worked with the Freedman's Bureau providing medical care for former slaves. She retired in 1880 and lived in Boston, where in 1883 she published her *Book of Medical Discourses,* which provided medical advice to help women care for themselves and their children.[19]

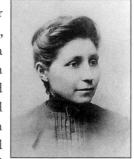

In 1889, Susan La Flesche graduated first in her class from the Woman's Medical College of Pennsylvania, becoming the first Native American woman to receive a medical degree. She interned at the Woman's Hospital in Philadelphia and worked as the government-appointed physician at the Omaha agency school and as medical missionary to her tribe on the Omaha Reservation in Nebraska, serving on behalf of the Women's National Indian Association. She married in 1894 and added her husband's name, Picotte, to her own. She spent her entire professional life improving the health conditions

Susan La Flesche Picotte, MD
[Nebraska State Historical Society, RG2026.PH6]

of the Omaha tribe, and in 1913, finally realized her dream when a hospital was established in Walthill, Nebraska. After her death from cancer, the hospital was renamed in her honor.[20]

MEDICAL COLLEGES FOR WOMEN

Through the mid- to late nineteenth century, most male physicians clung to the traditional arguments that women were too weak and lacking in intellectual capacity to practice medicine and warned that the traditional virtues of female modesty and chastity would be lost if women were permitted to study anatomy, especially male anatomy. At the same time, women's rights advocates and others argued that women physicians were essential to preserving women's health, as well as those traditional virtues, since they would permit women sufferers to seek medical treatment from members of their own sex. Because of the barriers against admitting women into existing medical schools, supporters of women in medicine saw a need to establish a medical school exclusively for females. In Boston, Samuel Gregory, MD, led a group of homeopathic physicians interested in teaching midwifery in opening the Boston Female Medical College in 1848. Initially the school taught only midwifery, but in 1850 the curriculum was expanded to become a full medical school. It was rechartered in 1856 as the New England Female Medical College and in 1873 the school merged with Boston University. The college remained homeopathic until after World War I when it became an allopathic college. On 12 October 1850, a group of Quaker businessmen, clergy, and physicians opened the Female Medical College of Pennsylvania, an allopathic medical school, in Philadelphia. The college graduated its first class, consisting of eight women, in December 1852. With the outbreak of the American Civil War, the school was forced to close, but in 1867, it reopened as the Woman's Medical College of Pennsylvania under the leadership of one of its first graduates, Ann Preston, MD.[21]

Inspired by the success of these first schools, between 1850 and 1895, a total of nineteen medical schools were founded exclusively for the training of female physicians. Unfortunately, some of these medical schools were underfunded or suffered from low enrollments and closed after only a couple of years. By 1904, sixteen of those nineteen female medical schools had closed,[22] leaving only the Woman's Medical College of Pennsylvania, the Woman's Medical College of Baltimore (closed in 1909), and the homeopathic New York Medical College and Hospital for Women (closed in 1918).[23]

In 1969, the Woman's Medical College of Pennsylvania, which at the time was the only remaining all-female medical college in the world, expanded into a coeducational institution, becoming the Medical College of Pennsylvania. In 1970, it merged with Hahnemann Medical College, and in 2002 the combined schools evolved into what is currently known as Drexel University College of Medicine.[24]

WOMEN IN OSTEOPATHIC MEDICINE

In contrast to the "regular" medical profession, women were welcomed into the DO profession from the very beginning. Dr. A.T. Still, founder of the osteopathic profession, strongly supported the right of women to be practitioners of the healing arts. The first class of the American School of Osteopathy in 1892 had six women enrolled. Five years later in 1897, Dr. Alice Patterson, one of the early faculty members, wrote, "We now have about one hundred earnest, intelligent, level headed, and rather strong-minded young women in our school."[25] During an age when women were regularly denied entrance into the majority of allopathic medical colleges, osteopathic medical schools openly welcomed female applicants. The first annual admissions catalogue for the American School of Osteopathy stated:

Women Received

Women are admitted on the same terms as men. It is the policy of the school that there shall be no distinction as to sex, and that all shall have the same opportunities, and be held to the same requirements. They pursue the same studies, attend the same lectures, are subjected to the same rules, and pass the same examinations. Separate reception rooms and all necessary facilities are provided for their comfort and enjoyment.[26]

By 1908, over 35 percent of all DOs in the country were women and by 1923, 50 percent of all osteopathic medical students in the United States were women.[27] This was quite an accomplishment considering that most of the few women physicians practicing in the country at the time had to attend schools dedicated solely to the training of female physicians. The early osteopathic colleges, on the other hand, not only allowed, but in fact encouraged the enrollment of women. The November 1896 journal of the Pacific College of Osteopathy in California stated, "The Science of osteopathy appeals to women who desire a noble, uplifting work,"[28] and in February 1897 the publication *Osteopath* stated, "A woman whose natural inclination is towards the benefit and assistance of the less fortunate of human kind, and who desires to allay herself with some work that while acting constantly as a moral uplift, will yet in an agreeable and rapid way place her peculiarly above all concern for the future, has the basis furnished her in osteopathy."[29] Dr. Still himself took note of the success of the female students: "The women have done well in the classes, clinics and practice and are as well worthy of diplomas as any gentleman."[30]

The women who managed to graduate from the allopathic, homeopathic, and eclectic medical schools still faced many struggles. Although their numbers were very slowly increasing, women were often not accorded equal treatment and consideration, especially by regular physicians. Female medical doctors found it difficult to obtain internships and hospital appointments. It was not until 1915 that the American Medical Association would finally admit female MDs as members of their organization. In contrast, women DOs had been members and officers in the American Osteopathic Association (AOA) since its founding in 1897 (called the American Association for the Advancement of Osteopathy until 1901), and many women actively participated in the formation of the association.[31] For fifty-two of the first fifty-six years of the AOA, there was at least one woman serving as a vice president (the organization has three vice presidents). Throughout this time, several women were nominated for president, but none were ever elected to this position until July 2009 when Karen Nichols, DO, became the first woman elected as president of the AOA.[32]

Inspired by the success of the new practice of osteopathy and of Dr. Still's osteopathic school, new osteopathic schools sprang up in Des Moines, Minneapolis, Milwaukee, Chicago, Denver, Boston, and in the states of North Dakota, Kentucky, Pennsylvania, and California. By 1900, there were about a dozen schools, but unfortunately not all of these schools met the high standards of the profession. The newly formed Associated Colleges of Osteopathy, in cooperation with the AOA's Committee on Education, set standards for curriculum and length of study to ensure professional standards in its member schools and attempted to shut down inferior diploma mills and phony correspondence schools.[33] By 1902 the osteopathic profession had recognized the need to increase the educational standards of the osteopathic schools. The newly organized AOA Committee on Education issued a report urging "the rapid establishment of a three-year course and the introduction of a four-year curriculum as soon as was practical."[34]

There are few statistics for the first decades of the twentieth century, but in the 1920s, female enrollment in both osteopathic and allopathic medical colleges began to decline. From an all-time high of 50 percent female enrollment in 1923, osteopathic female enrollment by 1928 had dropped to 12 percent.[35] This decline in female enrollment would continue for almost another decade until the late 1930s when it would start to increase again. At the same time, allopathic medical schools had proportionally few women graduates: 2.6 percent of 1909 graduates were women and 5.4 percent were women in 1927. After that the percentage decreased to about 5 percent and remained steady until 1940.[36]

There was also a disproportionate distribution of DOs throughout the country in the early twentieth century, attributable to the facts that DOs were denied staff privileges at allopathic hospitals and that the existing medical establishment had blocked the granting of full medical licenses to DOs in some states. Because of these barriers, DOs tended to aggregate around existing osteopathic hospitals in those states that permitted full practice rights, resulting in numerous areas of the country having little to no osteopathic presence. This dearth of osteopathic physicians in states with limited practice rights made it difficult for the profession to obtain enough momentum to get licensing legislation passed in those states.

The dynamic changed during World War II when many male physicians entered military service, increasing the demand for new physicians on the home front, and the percentage of women filling medical school slots swelled as men joined the armed forces. Internships and faculty appointments also became available for women in ever-increasing numbers during the war. However, in the late 1940s following the end of World War II, the return of men from the war and the GI Bill resulted in a dramatic reversal in female enrollments. This swing back towards male dominance of medicine not only continued, but actually increased during the 1950s and '60s. The percentage of women in medical schools dropped dramatically and some have referred to this decline as "the years of stagnation." In allopathic medical schools, unofficial quotas and the hostility of faculty and administration toward female students, perhaps due to male concerns about competition for jobs, combined with a general reluctance on the part of families to spend money educating women who society expected to marry and raise families, meant that the number of women seeking medical training decreased during the post–World War II years.[37]

In 1966, the United States had fewer women enrolled in medical schools than any other developed or developing countries.[38] As a reflection of this trend, the decades of the 1950s and 1960s were called the era of Putting Hubby Through. Many of the medical schools organized and actively encouraged student wives' organizations, which frequently awarded "Putting Hubby Through" certificates. In 1960, the Chicago College of Osteopathy referred to these certificates as "Pushing Hubby Through".[39] The presentations of these certificates were frequently likened to the wife receiving her PhT degree. Medical schools, both osteopathic and allopathic, were strongly dominated by men, and there was a general sentiment that a woman's role was to support her husband.

The osteopathic medical schools were no exception to the general trend of declining female enrollment after World War II. However, their female enrollment numbers hit their lowest point in 1964, while female enrollment in the allopathic schools continued to decline for another two years, hitting their low in 1966. Once again, osteopathic colleges led the way to increasing female enrollment when in 1965, two years before allopathic medical schools, enrollment numbers and percentages of female enrollment began the road to recovery.[40]

In 1964, only four women graduated from the five osteopathic colleges (1.1 percent of the total graduates), and the entire student body contained only twenty-eight female osteopathic medical students (1.8 percent). The following year, the number of females increased to 2.5 percent of the graduates and 2.3 percent of all osteopathic students.[41] The numbers and percentages of female DO students grew continuously from the late 1960s through the 1980s. In the 1970s and '80s, the enrollment rate of women entering medical schools alone increased by over 850 percent.[42] By 1990, 24.3 percent of the DO graduates and 24.4 percent of the total osteopathic students were female.[43] This swing of the pendulum continued, and female enrollment increased throughout the 1990s and into the early 2000s to arrive at the fifty-fifty male to female distributions now observed in most osteopathic medical schools.

As female enrollment increased in medical schools, not everyone was in lock-step agreement with the trend. There remained, and to a lesser degree still remains to this day, some chauvinistic individuals who steadfastly oppose this trend. Those opposed to large numbers of women attending medical schools frequently point

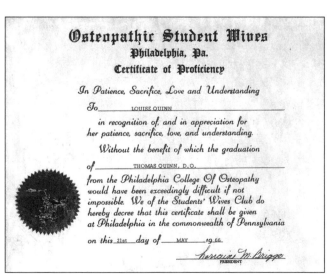

A typical Putting Hubby Through (PhT) Certificate awarded by the Philadelphia College of Osteopathy in 1966. [Sissy (Louise) Quinn]

Osteopathic Student Wives
Philadelphia, Pa.
Certificate of Proficiency

In Patience, Sacrifice, Love and Understanding

To _____ LOUISE QUINN _____

in recognition of, and in appreciation for her patience, sacrifice, love, and understanding.

Without the benefit of which the graduation

of _____ THOMAS QUINN, D.O. _____

from the Philadelphia College Of Osteopathy would have been exceedingly difficult if not impossible. We of the Students' Wives Club do hereby decree that this certificate shall be given at Philadelphia in the commonwealth of Pennsylvania

on this 21st day of _____ MAY _____ 19 66

_____ Lorraine M. Briggs _____
PRESIDENT

to studies that appear to demonstrate that women are much less likely than men to enter rural medical practice,[44] arguing that this contributes to the shortage of practicing physicians in rural areas. However, a more important cause of the shortage in rural physicians is overspecialization, which has led to a shortage of primary care physicians, who are more likely to establish a rural practice than a specialist. The osteopathic medical profession meanwhile has consistently provided a larger proportion of rural physicians. This can be attributed in part to the larger percentage of DOs who enter primary care medicine, and may also reflect the distinct trend for DOs to provide medical care to medically underserved communities.

Some opponents to women in medicine argue that more female physicians are needed to equal the work of male physicians. One study notes, "On average 87 percent of male doctors maintain a full-time medical practice whereas only 59 percent of female physicians maintain a full-time medical practice throughout their career."[45] These figures are used to show that the average female doctor will spend fewer years practicing than her male counterpart; however, not every female physician is average. These figures fail to show the large number of female physicians who maintain fully active practices throughout their entire professional careers. One example is Anne Wales, DO, who at 101 years of age was still teaching osteopathic manipulative techniques to other osteopathic physicians (see chapter 3).

It seems likely that the trend will continue towards higher female enrollment; it may even be that both the osteopathic and allopathic medical professions will become female-dominated in the future. In 2004, Geraldine O'Shea, DO, an internist and vice chair of the AOA Women's Health Advisory Committee, said, "A change is coming in the field of healthcare—there will be more women in leadership positions. The feet of women are marching towards medicine, and there's no way we can't break through doors—just because of sheer numbers."[46]

NOTES

1. Schiebinger, *The Mind Has No Sex?*, 2.

2. Schiebinger, *The Mind Has No Sex?*, 250–57; and Offen, *European Feminisms*, 43.

3. "James Barry," in *Oxford Dictionary of National Biography*, 1244–45; and Hacker, *Indomitable Lady Doctors*, 3–16.

4. Armstrong and Armstrong, *Great American Medicine Show*, 3, 24–30, quote at 3.

5. Kett, *Formation of the American Medical Profession*, 23.

6. There are many excellent works on the history of medicine in America and the history of women in medicine. A few examples are Duffy, *The Healers*; Rossiter, *Women Scientists in America*; Bonner, *To the Ends of the Earth*; Kirschmann, *A Vital Force*; Starr, *Social Transformation of American Medicine*; Morantz-Sanchez, *Sympathy and Science*; and Burbick, *Healing the Republic*.

7. Hanaford, *Daughters of America,* 556.

8. Hunt, *Glances and Glimpses,* 123.

9. Simpson and Weiser, "Studying the Impact of Women on Osteopathic Physician Workforce Predictions," *JAOA* 96, no. 2 (Feb. 1996): 107.

10. Heffel, *Opportunities in Osteopathic Medicine Today,* 42–43.

11. Walter, *Women and Osteopathic Medicine,* 18–19; and Roberta Hobson and Susan E. Cayleff, "Harriot Kezia Hunt," in *American National Biography,* 11:490–91.

12. Duffy, *The Healers,* 3.

13. Ibid., 271–72.

14. Ibid., 271–72; and Regina Markell Morantz-Sanchez, "Elizabeth Blackwell," in *American National Biography,* 2:892–94.

15. Duffy, *The Healers,* 272; and Regina Markell Morantz-Sanchez, "Elizabeth Blackwell," in *American National Biography,* 2:892–94.

16. Schiebinger, *The Mind Has No Sex?,* 7–8; Duffy, *The Healers,* 272–73; and Regina Markell Morantz-Sanchez, "Elizabeth Blackwell," in *American National Biography,* 2:892–94.

17. Bynum, *Western Medical Tradition,* 147.

18. Sarah K. A. Pfatteicher, "Rebecca Davis Lee Crumpler," in *American National Biography,* 5:823–25.

19. Crumpler, *Book of Medical Discourses,* 1–4; and Sarah K. A. Pfatteicher, "Rebecca Davis Lee Crumpler," in *American National Biography,* 5:823–25. Also see "Outstanding Women Doctors: They Make Their Mark in Medicine," *Ebony,* May 1964, 68–76.

20. Peggy Pascoe, "Susan La Flesche Picotte," in *American National Biography,* 17:487–88.

21. Duffy, *The Healers,* 273; and Bonner, *To the Ends of the Earth,* 138–59.

22. Duffy, *The Healers,* 176–77.

23. *Flexner Report* (1910), 178.

24. Drexel University College of Medicine, "History, 1848–2002," accessed 17 Feb. 2011, http://www.drexelmed.edu/Home/AboutTheCollege/History.aspx.

25. Patterson, "Women in Osteopathy," *Journal of Osteopathy* 4, no. 2 (June 1897): 71–72.

26. *Catalogue of the American School of Osteopathy, Kirksville, Missouri, 1897–98,* 52, MOM.

27. Walter, *Women and Osteopathic Medicine,* 15, 20–21.

28. "A Noble Life-Work," *Journal of Osteopathy* 3, no. 5 (Nov. 1896): 3.

29. "The Science of Osteopathy," *The Osteopath* 1 (Feb. 1897): 4.

30. Still, *Autobiography,* 133.

31. Booth, *History of Osteopathy,* 251–60.

32. Fitzgerald, "Women in History, Pioneers of the Profession," *The DO* 25 (Dec. 1984): 68; and *AOA Daily Report,* 19 July 2009.

33. American Osteopathic Association, *History of Osteopathic Medicine Virtual Museum,* accessed 17 Feb. 2011, http://history.osteopathic.org/.

34. Booth, *History of Osteopathy,* 269.

35. Walter, *Women and Osteopathic Medicine,* 20–21.

36. Duffy, *The Healers,* 277.

37. Walter, *Women and Osteopathic Medicine,* 21–22; and Duffy, *The Healers,* 277.

38. Duffy, *The Healers,* 36.

39. "Chicago Wives Honored for 'Pushing Hubby Through,'" *Forum of Osteopathy* 34 (July 1960): 46.

40. *AOA Fact Sheet, 1967.*

41. *AOA Yearbook and Directory, 1979–80*, 308.

42. McNiven, "Women in Medicine," *Michigan Medicine* (Sept. 1991): 34.

43. *AOA Fact Sheet*, 1991.

44. Rosenblatt, "Which Medical Schools Produce Rural Physicians?" *JAMA* 268, no. 12 (Sept. 1992): 1559–65.

45. Heins et al., "Special Communication: Comparison of Productivity of Women and Men Physicians," *JAMA* 237, no. 23 (June 1977): 2514–17, quote at 2514.

46. Greenfield, "Women Wielding Influence," *The DO* 45 (Dec. 2004): 29.

Chapter Two

Women and the Founding of Osteopathic Medicine

"I opened wide the doors of my first school for ladies.... Why not elevate our sister's mentality, qualify her to fill all places of trust and honor, place her hand and head with the skilled arts?"

Andrew Taylor Still, MD, DO

"... the firm hand of the woman osteopathist is none the less effectual on account of her sex."

Alice Patterson, DO

MEDICAL PRACTITIONERS OF THE MID-NINETEENTH CENTURY were poorly trained compared to physicians today. They had little understanding of the true causes of disease and many of their treatments were prescientific and crude at best. It was not until 1857 when French microbiologist Louis Pasteur published his first scientific paper on germ theory[1] that a scientist had put forward the idea that common diseases were caused by specific germs. Joseph Lister, influenced by Pasteur's discoveries, studied infections from injuries and pioneered the use of antiseptics to kill germs during surgery, greatly reducing postoperative mortality. In the 1870s, Robert Koch was the first to prove a causal relationship between a bacillus and a disease when he isolated the anthrax bacillus and developed an inoculation; he later isolated the bacilli responsible for cholera and tuberculosis. Through the work of researchers such as Pasteur, Koch, and Lister, scientists began to understand the microbiological basis of disease, although it took generations for their theories to be fully accepted by the scientific community.

Before these scientific discoveries, medical treatments were based on the assumption that illness was caused by an imbalance in bodily humors, and many medical treatments thought to restore the balance were dangerous. Bloodletting, laxatives, purgatives, narcotics, alcohol, arsenic, and mercury compounds were freely administered, often to the detriment of the patient. These drastic forms of treatment are often called "heroic medicine" and more often than not, the patient would have had a better chance of surviving if they had not been treated by a physician at all. In an 1860 address to the Massachusetts Medical Society, Oliver Wendell Holmes Sr., MD, said, "I firmly believe that if the whole *materia medica*, as now used, could be sunk to the bottom of the sea, it would be all the better for mankind—and all the worse for the fishes."[2]

A century earlier, Benjamin Rush, a prominent Philadelphia physician who had studied medicine in Philadelphia and earned a medical degree from the University of Edinburgh, was a strong proponent of this form of treatment. After earning his medical degree in England, Rush opened a practice in Philadelphia and taught chemistry at the College of Philadelphia; he also served in the Second Continental Congress, where he signed the Declaration of Independence, and briefly served as surgeon general in the Continental army. In addition to an active medical career, Rush was involved in moral and humanitarian reforms, advocating for education, prison reform, temperance, abolition of slavery, and elimination of tobacco, as well as promoting fresh air and personal hygiene to maintain health. After the war, he was on the staff of the Philadelphia Hospital and was professor of medical theory and clinical practice at the University of Pennsylvania, despite his attachment to medical treatments that were even then considered somewhat old-fashioned. Dr. Rush became even more enthusiastic about these treatments after a series of coincidental successes during the yellow fever epidemic of 1793 led him to formulate the idea of the unity of disease—that all diseases were caused by tension in the blood vessels, which could be relieved by purging and bleeding. Even some of his contemporaries felt that Rush was excessive in his use of bloodletting. William Cobbett, a British journalist, accused Rush of killing more patients than he saved. Rush sued him for libel. After losing the case, Cobbett returned to England in 1800, probably to avoid punishment.[3] Ironically, only a year earlier, George Washington had died of causes now attributed to heroic medicine. In December 1799 Washington was suffering from a throat infection and was attended by three regular physicians. They blistered his skin and applied poultices of wheat bran to his legs and feet; a purgative of mercury (calomel) left him weak and dehydrated. The physicians also bled Washington four times in less than a twenty-four hour period—each time he became progressively weaker. Modern medical experts believe that the combination of mercury poisoning and excessive bloodletting was the direct cause of Washington's death, and that he probably would have survived if the physicians had not been called.[4]

When Andrew Taylor Still was born, most of these treatments were still commonly used, but the popular health movement was underway and other forms of medical practice were developing. Many of those new types of medicine were short-lived, but their popularity no doubt influenced the young doctor.

ANDREW TAYLOR STILL AND THE ORIGINS OF OSTEOPATHY

Andrew Taylor Still was born in Lee County, Virginia, the third of nine children of Rev. Abraham (Abram) and Martha Still. In addition to being a circuit rider for the Methodist Church, Abram Still was, as Andrew Still described him, "a man educated to do all kinds of work,...a minister, doctor, farmer, and a practical millwright."[5] It was common for Methodist ministers to also practice medicine, both to supplement their income and to minister to the physical as well as the spiritual needs of their flocks. Frontier doctors often relied on botanical remedies, but Rev. Still also used the traditional heroic treatments that Dr. Henry Wilkens included in his new version of John Wesley's medical manual, an edition widely used by Methodist circuit riders.[6]

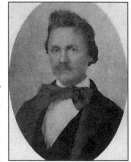

Andrew T. Still, MD, 1850
[MOM 1997.04.219]

Andrew Still studied medicine and apprenticed with his father, probably beginning in the 1840s when the family was living in Missouri. Dr. A. T. Still stated that he attended the Kansas City College of Physicians and Surgeons during the winter of 1865/66, but did not return to receive his diploma. Dr. Still's formal training cannot be verified, but we do know that he learned his craft primarily through self-study, apprenticeship, and practical experience. In his autobiography, Still writes of studying anatomy "from the great book of nature," learning about muscles, bones, and nerves while skinning animals he had hunted. In the 1850s, while living in Kansas and practicing medicine with his father among the Shawnee at the Wakarusa Mission, where the church had sent Abram Still, Andrew Still "became a robber in the name of science. Indian graves were desecrated and the bodies of the sleeping dead exhumed in the name of science...and [I] studied the dead that the living might be benefited."[7]

In the years leading up to the Civil War, the Still family sided with the abolitionists, and Andrew became involved in the border skirmishes and political wrangling that led up to Kansas eventually joining the Union as a free state. Andrew Still served in an abolitionist militia before the war, but also counted members of proslavery families among his patients.

A. T. Still served as a scout surgeon under General John C. Fremont in 1853 and was involved in the skirmishes between Kansans and Missourians in the fight to have Kansas join the Union as a free state. The Still brothers, including Andrew, were friends with John Brown and allied with him in the fight against the effort to make Kansas a slave state. In 1857, Dr. Andrew Still was elected to the Free Kansas legislature.[8]

When the Civil War broke out, Still joined the 9th Kansas Cavalry, where he served as a medical officer; he later wrote that, "a surgeon's outfit was complete when it contained calomel, quinine, whiskey, opium, rags, and a knife. If a patient had one foot in the grave and a half-pint of whiskey in the bottle, the doctor would work as hard to get the whiskey out of the bottle as to keep the foot from the grave." When his unit was disbanded in 1862, Still returned to his home state and organized a company of Kansas volunteers. His company was assigned to patrol the Santa Fe Trail as it ran across Douglas County, Kansas. During the war he was promoted from captain to major. Dr. Still's experience as a surgeon during the Civil War further eroded his confidence in the medications and treatments being used at the time. In his autobiography, he wrote of seeing doctors dose sick or injured men with liquor and opium that did little or nothing to treat their ailments and often created addicts and drunks. He also noted that, "I began to see during the civil war, in that part of the states of Missouri and Kansas where the doctors were shut out, the children did not die."[9]

Other, more personal experiences further eroded Still's faith in traditional medical practices. In 1849, Andrew had married Mary Margaret Vaughn, of whom he wrote in his autobiography, "She was to me beautiful, kind, active, and abounded in love and good sense. She loved God and all His Ways."[10] Together they moved to the Wakarusa Reservation where they had a farm and Mary Margaret taught in the mission school, while around them the disputes that would lead to the Civil War played out in the border wars known as Bleeding Kansas. Andrew's sister Marovia later recalled "We seemed to live on excitement in those days," keeping a watch for marauders and preparing for battle.[11]

Their first child, Marusha, was born in 1849, and Abraham was born in 1852. Then in 1855, Andrew and Mary Margaret mourned the death of an infant son. Another daughter, Susan, was born in 1856. Mary Margaret died in 1859, shortly after giving birth to their fifth child, a son who lived only six days. Andrew Still wrote in his autobiography, "Then my wife, who had shared my misfortunes, trials, and sorrows, …soared to that world of love and glory for which she had lived all her life."[12]

A year later, Still married Mary Elvira Turner, a schoolteacher and daughter of a pharmacist from New York, whom he met while she was living with her sister in Edgerton, Kansas, near the Wakarusa Reservation.[13] Mary Elvira had attended Poughkeepsie Female Seminary and had helped her father run his small pharmacy, where she had learned a good deal about sickness and the compounding of drugs. On many occasions, she opined that if only women could be doctors she would surely have entered that profession.[14] Because of her knowledge of sickness and her experience in her father's pharmacy, Mary Elvira was asked to examine a neighbor's sick chil-

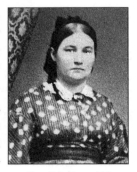

Mary Elvira Turner Still (second wife of A. T. Still) [Courtesy of Martha Wadlin]

dren. Physicians were scarce on the frontier, so women like Mary Elvira were valued for their skills and knowledge. After examining the girls, Mary Elvira advised the mother that the children might have scarlet fever and she should call for a physician. That physician was Andrew T. Still, MD.

Mary Elvira was not initially impressed by the widower with four children, but during an epidemic of scarlet fever in the spring of 1860, Dr. Still made frequent visits to patients in Edgerton and called on Mary Elvira. Their love blossomed, but Mary refused to marry Andrew Still until he promised to give up chewing tobacco. The Stills' first child, a son, was born in 1861, shortly after Andrew had enlisted as a medical officer in the Union army, but lived only fifty-four days. A daughter, Marcia Ione Still, was born in 1863. Other children would follow: Charles in 1865, twins Herman and Harry in 1867, Fred in 1874, and Blanche in 1876.

In 1864, just months after Still had been discharged from the army, the couple lost three children (Abraham, Susan, and an adopted daughter) to a meningitis epidemic, and just four weeks later, their daughter Marcia died of pneumonia. He wrote, "War had left my family unharmed; but when the dark wings of spinal meningitis hovered over the land, it seemed to select my loved ones for its prey."[15] The doctor's standard treatments could do nothing to help, and he blamed "gross ignorance on the part of the medical profession." Although Dr. Still had previously questioned the usefulness of many traditional medical practices,[16] it would take the devastating loss of four children to drive him to present his most critical challenge to orthodox medicine. He felt confident that there were better and less toxic methods of treatment.

START OF A NEW SCIENCE

In his autobiography, Andrew Still declared that on 22 June 1874 he completely severed his ties with mainstream medicine, and "I flung to the breeze the banner of Osteopathy."[17] But in 1874, his new science did not yet have a name. It was not until 1889, when he was considering the need for a school to teach the new science, that he bothered to give it a name. He chose osteopathy from *osteon*, meaning "bone," and *pathos*, meaning "to suffer." Immediately his son Charles protested that the word was not in the dictionary. Dr Still replied, "I know it; we are going to put it there."[18]

The years leading up to 1874 were devoted to searching for ways to improve the practice of medicine, and in particular, to find a cure for the spinal meningitis that had devastated his family. During this time, Dr. Still apparently became increasingly interested in what was known as bonesetting, a form of manipulative practice limited to the field of orthopedics. He likely felt that by learning these techniques he would be able to treat a wider range of disorders and be better equipped to treat the whole person. Bonesetting was a talent usually passed down from one family member to another, and practitioners were not a respected group of healers. In addition to reducing dislocations, they also manipulated painful and diseased joints, based on the idea that they were caused by "a bone out of place." Their diagnoses were crude, limited, and not accepted by organized medicine. As Dr. Still practiced this form of therapy however, he discovered that the sudden flexion and extension procedures used by bonesetters were not beneficial to orthopedic problems alone.[19] After years of investigation and clinical observation, Dr. Still found that manipulative therapy techniques could "alleviate painful and distressing symptoms of disease and injury by mechanical displacement of fluids, removal of toxic materials, inducing neurovascular and neuromuscular effects, thus producing metabolic, biochemical, and circulatory changes."[20] Dr. Still stated, "I found mechanical causes for disordered functioning."[21]

In 1991, Charles E. Still Jr., grandson of A. T. Still, published *Frontier Doctor, Medical Pioneer*, in which he gives a different story. He states that his grandfather never studied bonesetting. He writes that in the early years of osteopathy, when Dr. Still first began refusing to use his MD designation but had not yet given his new science a name, patients noted the similarities between the therapy his grandfather had developed independently and the treatments given by the bonesetters. Since they had no other designation or title to give him, they started calling Dr. Andrew Still a "Lightening Bone Setter."[22] The Museum of Osteopathic Medicine (formerly Still National Osteopathic Museum) has an early business card from Still's time in Kirksville on which the doctor himself used this designation, possibly because it would have been familiar to potential patients. It is likely that we will never know the level of Dr. Still's involvement with bonesetting since he does not mention it in his autobiography and there are no other known records to indicate his involvement with this form of treatment.[23]

As Andrew Still continued to study the workings of the human body and struggled to articulate his growing sense of the body's natural ability to heal itself, his ideas were met with rejection and attacks on his medical reputation. Many of Dr. Still's family, friends, and professional colleagues were shocked by his total rejection of regular medicine. Other doctors in the area considered his new concepts to be "sheer lunacy," and most of the local population shared the same sentiment.[24] Even members of his own family urged him to give up his odd ideas and return to practicing traditional medicine. He explored magnetism, physiomedicalism, mesmerism (hypnosis), Thomsonianism, and phrenology. His exploration of Spiritualism and evolutionary theories led to a local preacher denouncing him as sacrilegious, and Baker University, which his family had helped to found, quickly and bluntly refused his proposal to teach osteopathy at the school. Dr. Still's initial intention was to incorporate his theories into mainstream medicine, but the mainstream medical community rejected his ideas about the uselessness of traditional drugs and treatments, and the efficacy of manipulation to alleviate the mechanical causes of illness and restore the body's natural ability to heal itself. His ideas were ridiculed and he was ostracized.[25] Had he been allowed to present his theories to the medical community and had they been accepted, osteopathic medicine as we know it today would not exist.

Rejected in Kansas, Dr. Still moved to Macon County, Missouri, in 1874, with the hope of joining the medical practice of his brother Edward C. Still, MD. Mary Elvira and Andrew Still had by this time started a new family, but his family remained in Kansas; they were to join him as soon as he was established. Upon arriving in Macon, Andrew discovered that his brother suffered from morphine addiction, which was not uncommon due to the frequent prescription of this drug by orthodox physicians at the time. Andrew stayed for three months to help Edward with his addiction.[26] Edward, however, would not accept him into his medical practice because he felt that Andrew would ruin his business with his unorthodox practice of adjusting people to treat their illnesses. He also complained that Andrew simply did not look like a professional physician due to the way he dressed and behaved.[27] At first Andrew could not understand why Edward would not help. Only later, when he found a letter from their brother James, also an MD, warning Edward that

"[Andrew] was crazy, had lost his mind and supply of truth-loving manhood,"[28] did he fully understand Edward's reluctance to help. Years later, after Andrew became successful and opened the American School of Osteopathy, Edward enrolled in the first class and became an osteopath in 1894. His brother James soon followed, enrolling one year after Edward and graduating in 1895.[29]

Determined to succeed, Andrew opened his own practice in Macon. Months passed and Andrew still struggled to establish himself. He saw only a few patients and remained practically unknown. Most of the patients he did treat had muscle and joint injuries and so it remained unnoticed that, unlike orthodox physicians, he used few medications. Some patients who Edward was not successful in treating came instead to Andrew and responded well to his new treatment.[30] Andrew's fortunes quickly changed when Macon was hit with an epidemic of bloody flux, a form of acute bloody diarrhea with a particularly high mortality rate among the children and elderly. Andrew Still initially offered his services to several poor families who could not afford to pay a physician, but his manipulative treatments produced such spectacular success that his office was soon packed with paying patients.[31]

After the epidemic waned, Dr. Still again became a victim of his own accomplishments. Though he had remarkable outcomes in fighting the epidemic of bloody flux, the town began to abound with rumors about his extraordinary successes. Realizing that he produced results largely without the use of medications, some people mistakenly believed him to possess supernatural powers and the ability to expel demons with his hands. It was not long before the religious community of Macon ostracized him for his unorthodox methods. One minister decried the doctor as a "hopeless sinner" and another accused him of being "possessed by the devil."[32] People began to avoid him on the streets, considering him to be some kind of "strange creature." Faced with such condemnation, Andrew Still again went searching for a community where he could practice his new form of medicine.[33]

Dr. Still moved to Kirksville, Missouri, a little over thirty miles north of Macon, in February 1875. He had misgivings that the negative rumors would travel to Kirksville from nearby Macon, but Kirksville was a small town, the citizens were friendly, and the medical community was apparently not opposed to newcomers. The presence of an active Spiritualist society in town may have helped, and some prominent citizens were interested in new philosophies. Several people offered to help him get established. Julia Ivie, owner of a local hotel, allowed Dr. Still to stay there for free until he established his practice. Charlie Chinn gave him free office space until he was able to start payments. Dr. F. A. Grove, Judge Linder, and Robert

Harris all assisted the new physician until his practice was established. In May 1875, his wife and their four children moved to Kirksville to be with him.[34]

During the early years, Andrew Still's practice in Kirksville remained small, so he traveled to other towns looking for patients in order to earn enough to support his growing family. While traveling around, Dr. Still gave lectures and demonstrations to promote his new ideas.[355] He often began his lectures with a prayer. The prayer he delivered on 4 July 1891, in Hannibal, Missouri, combined the Lord's Prayer with humor, temperance, distrust for medications, and a little osteopathy.

> Our Father, who art in Heaven and in Earth and in all things but whiskey and such things as men have no business with, thou hast been asked to take the place of father by us, give us our daily bread, and no whiskey; give us reason and keep snakes out of our boots. Give us good knowledge of our true bodily forms and tell us how to know when a bone has strayed from its true position and how to return them to their natural places. Also lead us not into temptations to get drunk when our limbs are on a strain and make a few pains, but teach us how to cure or stop fever, mumps, measles, flux and all disease of the seasons as they roll around. Thou knowest our people do foolish things when they are sick. O, Lord throw a few lightning bugs of reason on our MDs. Thou knowest their eyes cannot all open at once like a litter of puppies but light them out one at a time, and if this failest open the minds of the people, so they will not be subjects of experiments any longer. And deliver us from all drugs, for thou seeth just in front of us a world of maniacs, idiots, criminals, nakedness for the babies and hunger for the mothers. For thine is the kingdom from now on.
> Amen[366]

According to Dr. Homer E. Bailey, a medical historian, Dr. Still was always rejected by the medical community as a cultist, and regarded by the general public as an "eccentric genius" or a "deranged old man."[377] Still was known to carry human bones with him, which he would pull out to show his patients what he was going to do and what effect it would have on them.[388] In many cases, the only patients who would seek his care were those whose cases had been declared hopeless by orthodox physicians. In many cases, their conditions were indeed hopeless and the patients could not be helped. But there were also many whose conditions did respond to Dr. Still's new form of treatment. Harry Still described one such case:

> The lady had been in the [insane] asylum for several years. It seemed she had lost her mind suddenly while playing a piano. Father examined her

neck and found a lesion of the atlas (1st cervical vertebrae). In less time than I have taken in telling, the girl was as rational as ever. Strange to say, the first thing she said was "where is my piano and music?" She was anxious to finish the piece she had started playing three years before.[39]

The medical accuracy of this story could be questioned, since at the time Harry had no formal training as a physician and was acting only as an assistant to his father; however, it appears that the patient received dramatic relief from her symptoms.

By the mid-1880s, Dr. Still's reputation started to improve in the towns he visited. Patients lined up waiting for Dr. Still to arrive, in some cases, traveling long distances to be treated.[40] Osteopathy received newspaper publicity for the first time when Dr. Charles Still, son of A. T. Still and a recent graduate of the new osteopathic school, was asked to treat a seventeen-year-old girl. She had been competing in a high-kicking contest when she dislocated her hip and became unable to stand on that leg. Her parents took her to one of the more renowned surgeons in the city who, only four hours after the injury, diagnosed her with a tuberculosis condition of the hip. He treated the girl for five or six weeks without any success. The girl's father had already heard of the senior Dr. Still's success with osteopathy in Kirksville and learned that Dr. Charles Still was seeing patients in Kansas City. When he brought his daughter to the younger Dr. Still, her hips, thighs, and legs were bound with adhesive tape, she had an extension brace on her leg, and was walking with crutches. Because he was a newly graduated DO and the surgeon was one of the best-known physicians in Kansas City, Charles asked his father to examine the patient. After a thorough examination, Dr. A. T. Still diagnosed the condition as a dislocated hip and with his son's assistance, manipu-lated the hip, returning the head of the thigh bone to the hip socket. Dr. Still then said to the girl, "Young woman, you can walk." She immediately replied, "Oh no, Dr. Still, I can't walk." After some coaxing, the girl stepped on the leg and much to her surprise, she was able to walk.[41]

Under normal circumstances, the case would not have received publicity, but a newly established newspaper in Kansas City had instructed its reporters to be on the lookout for unusual news stories. After the eminent surgeon read of the girl's cure, he sent her father a hefty bill for services rendered. The father refused to pay the bill and the surgeon sued him. After waiting several months to make sure the osteopathic cure was permanent, the father countersued the surgeon for damages resulting from misdiagnosis and malpractice. Both suits were eventually dropped, but in the meantime, Dr. Still and osteopathy received much positive publicity.[42]

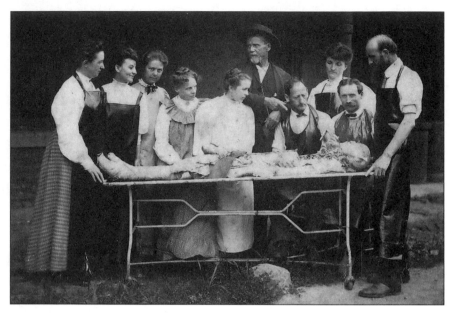

Open-air anatomy class with A. T. Still, 1898. [MOM PIC-DIS-3]

Dr. A. T. Still's fortunes in Kirksville changed in 1886 after he treated the young daughter of J. B. Mitchell, the town's highly influential Presbyterian minister. The girl had lost her ability to walk after falling off of a horse, and repeated efforts by other physicians had no effect. Dr. Still was called in as a last resort. With just one treatment, Dr. Still restored the full function of her legs. The grateful father praised Dr. Still and he was quickly accepted in local society.[43] By 1887, Dr. Still had set up a permanent office in his home in Kirksville. When his patient load increased so that he found it necessary to treat patients on the porch and even in the yard, he purchased a small cottage that he used for additional treatment rooms. Andrew Still's sons Charles and Harry worked as his assistants, but since they were not fully trained in the science of osteopathy, they were of limited help. The practice continued to grow and Dr. Still purchased another cottage to use as a waiting room and additional treatment rooms. The three small buildings gave Dr. Still and his sons a total of ten treatment rooms. By 1891, patients were traveling to Kirksville from throughout the country to be treated by Dr. Still and it was obvious that he would need more and better trained assistants if he had any hope of keeping up with the growing demand for his new form of treatment. That year he formed an informal class to prepare qualified "operators" to act as assistants at the infirmary and as instructors at the school he was planning to open.[44] This class included three of his sons, his daughter Blanche, Joe Hutten, William Wilderson, and Marcus L. Ward. Including Marcus Ward in this class proved to be a mistake. Only a few years later, Ward opened a competing osteopathic college just walking distance from Dr. Still's school and claimed that he (Ward), not Dr. Still, was the founder of osteopathy.[45]

Unexpected support for the new science of osteopathy came in June 1892, when Dr. William Smith, a graduate of the prestigious medical school at the University of Edinburgh was traveling throughout the United States demonstrating and selling surgical instruments. While traveling in Missouri, he heard patients praising Dr. Still and physicians complaining about losing patients to the old quack who was curing their patients without surgery. Dr. Smith decided to investigate for himself, so he traveled to Kirksville where he met Dr. Still and observed the results of his treatments; he was soon convinced and asked Dr. Still to teach him everything he knew. In return, Dr. Smith agreed to teach anatomy at the new medical school Dr. Still was considering.[46] Finally, A. T. Still had the expertise he needed to open the American School of Osteopathy (ASO). The school's original charter of May 1892, gave it the right to confer the doctor of medicine (MD) degree,[47] but Dr. Still felt this degree did not adequately reflect the training that the students received and instead made the fateful decision to confer the diplomate of osteopathy (DO) degree (later changed to doctor of osteopathy and currently doctor of osteopathic medicine). The original faculty consisted of Andrew Taylor Still and William Smith, who began his osteopathic studies before the school officially opened and received a hand-printed DO diploma signed by A. T. Still in February 1893. Both Dr. Still and Dr. Smith had been trained as orthodox physicians and were skilled in the use of drugs and surgery. Dr. Smith was also a trained anatomist. Their goal was not to replace the current system of medical care but to improve it.[48] Although Dr. Still's methods consisted primarily of his new science of osteopathy, the school did not teach only manipulative therapy. In a 1902 article, Dr. Still explained:

> The osteopathic concept includes surgery, which osteopathic physicians practice or recommend when it is indicated. Surgery is taught in all the osteopathic colleges. Osteopathy is not a drugless therapy.... It uses drugs, which have specific scientific value, such as antiseptics, parasiticides, antidotes, anesthetics or narcotics for the temporary relief of suffering....[49]

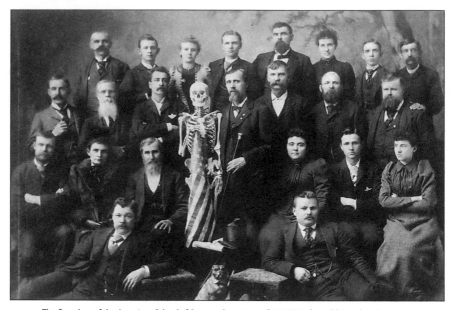

The first class of the American School of Osteopathy, winter of 1892/93 after additional students were added. The skinny fellow between William Smith (center left) and A. T. Still (center right) is "Columbus" the skeleton. [MOM 2007.09.01]

In his autobiography and other writings, however, A. T. Still and other early osteopaths frequently referred to themselves as drugless practitioners. In some cases, they condemned drugs, but indicated that they used anesthetics, antiseptics, and other drugs that had been proven effective. As the quality and effectiveness of medications have improved with the advancement of medical science in the twentieth and twenty-first centuries, modern osteopathic physicians have increased their use of these better-quality medications.

An early student of osteopathy was instrumental in the founding of another new medical technique—chiropractic. Both osteopathy and chiropractic utilize manipulative treatments, and it is believed that the originator of chiropractic learned about these techniques from a student who attended the ASO; however, these two medical practices have unique qualities that set them apart. Andrew Still wrote that "Osteopathy is based on the perfection of Nature's work. When all parts of the human body are in line we have health. When they are not the effect is disease. When the parts are readjusted disease gives place to health. The work of the osteopath is to adjust the body from the abnormal to the normal; then the abnormal condition gives place to the normal and health is the result of the normal condition."[50] Daniel David Palmer wrote that chiropractic was the art of "relieving abnormal conditions by adjusting displaced bones,"[51] but his techniques focused on adjusting the tension placed on the nerves by the vertebrae. According to the American Chiropractic Association "Chiropractic is a drug-free, hands-on approach to health care."[52] In contrast, osteopathic medicine from its inception has never been completely drug free. Surgery, obstetrics, less toxic medications, manipulation, and all other proven medical practices have always been part of osteopathic treatments as taught in American osteopathic medical schools.

Chiropractic was founded in 1897 when Daniel David Palmer opened the Palmer School of Magnetic Cure in Davenport, Iowa. In 1904, he changed the name of the school to the Palmer School of Chiropractic. According to Arthur G. Hildreth, DO, a member of the first class of the ASO, Palmer had learned about manipulative therapy from an osteopathic medical student by the name of J. Strother from Davenport, Iowa, who was one of Hildreth's classmates in the first class at the ASO. There is no evidence, however, that Strother ever graduated from the ASO or received a DO degree.[53] Dr. Hildreth also wrote that Mr. Palmer had received osteopathic treatments from Dr. A. T. Still for several weeks in the summer of 1893 and had dined with Dr. Still.

> When we next heard of him [Palmer], he had discovered a method of treating disease by the hands, which he called chiropractic...the Palmer method was along the line practiced by Dr. Still for a number of years before opening his school in 1892 at Kirksville, only it was a very crude and very poor imitation of the kind of manipulative therapy Dr. Still practiced.... Dr. Still was using manipulative methods for the alleviation of pain and suffering years before the man from Davenport was ever heard of.[54]

Dr. Alva A. Gregory, a close associate of Palmer and president of the Palmer-Gregory Chiropractic College in Oklahoma City, wrote in his 1910 *Spinal Treatment*,

> The first school that used the spinal thrust exclusively as a system for the treatment of all ailments, both acute and chronic, was started by D. D. Palmer, who obtained his first ideas of spinal lesions from an osteopath by the name of Struther.... We find no evidence whatever that he [D. D. Palmer] was a discoverer, but find facts to the contrary. Palmer being an uneducated man it has fallen to the hands of others to develop this science.[55]

While some scholars may debate the philosophical similarities between the two forms of treatment and the source of Palmer's ideas, any knowledgeable medical historian can verify that neither Still nor Palmer originated the idea of manipulation. The oldest known historic mention of manipulation of a vertebra can be traced to an ancient surgical manuscript dating from ancient Egypt (ca. 2800 BCE) at Giza.[56] Manipulation was also recorded in the Kong Fu writings (ca. 2650 BCE), and in the medical writings of Hippocrates (ca. 460–ca. 377 BCE) and Galen (129–ca. 199 CE). The most widely used form of manipulation in the era immediately before Still and Palmer was known as bonesetting, which can be traced back at least to the middle ages and likely influenced both men in developing their practices.

When osteopathic physicians first appeared on the scene in the latter part of the eighteenth century, there were already allopathic, homeopathic, eclectic, and even the little-known physiomedical physicians, all of whom identified themselves by the MD degree. The first osteopathic medical school immediately manifested its difference, not only by rejecting the MD degree and granting a previously unknown DO degree, but also by becoming the first medical school in America to open as a coeducational institution. From the first day of classes, women were accepted into osteopathic medicine on a completely equal basis with men.

WOMEN OF THE FIRST CLASS, 1894

At the time Dr. Still opened the ASO in October 1892, there were over one hundred medical schools (both regular and irregular) in the United States that offered MD degrees. Of these, sixty-eight accepted only male students, thirty-two accepted women (although not on equal terms), and five accepted exclusively female students. The ASO accepted men and women on equal terms, based on Dr. Still's strong belief in the equality of the sexes. In fact, a policy of giving tuition abatements to women suggests a preference to the female students. The first year, tuition was five hundred dollars for a man, but two hundred dollars for a woman.[57]

In 1893, the Johns Hopkins University School of Medicine opened in Baltimore, Maryland. It was originally planned to be an all-male school until a group of prominent Baltimore women offered the school a grant of $500,000 on the condition that the school accept women. This was an enormous sum in 1893, so the school agreed and the Johns Hopkins School of Medicine became coeducational. Other schools soon followed the lead of these two schools. As more medical schools became coeducational, the separate women's medical schools began to close; by 1904 there were only three still operating.[58]

On 4 October 1892, ten or eleven students arrived for the first day of classes in the newly established ASO,[59] which at that time was located in a small school-house. Six of the male students had previously earned MD degrees (four were allopathic MDs and two were homeopathic MDs), but none of the female students had preexisting MD degrees, although at least one had a college degree. Several additional students joined the class later; the class picture taken in the winter of 1892/93 showed twenty-one students, including five women. A sixth woman, Lou J. Kern (Meitz), was in the first class, but does not appear in this picture. Four of these women completed the program; Nettie Bolles, Lou Kern, Mamie Harter, and Blanche Still received their degrees and went on to practice osteopathic medicine. Annie Peters and J. Gentry did not complete their degrees, for reasons that are not recorded. These first female DOs were only the beginning. By 1908, over 35 percent of all DOs in the country were women, and by 1923, 50 percent of all osteopathic medical students in the United States were women.[60]

Jeanette "Nettie" Hubbard Bolles, DO

As a young woman, Jeanette (Nettie) Hubbard had witnessed the benefits of osteopathic medicine firsthand. During the border skirmishes of the 1850s, her father was seriously wounded and left for dead. The family called for their neighbor, Dr. Andrew Still, who removed the bullet and restored Nettie's father to health. Years later when Nettie's mother became paralyzed from a fall, she brought her to Kirksville to be treated by Dr. Still. Nettie was so impressed by the results of Dr. Still's treatments that she asked if she could study to become an osteopath; Nettie had already graduated from the University of Kansas. Dr. Still assured her that she could learn osteopathy the same as any man.[61]

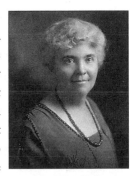

Jeanette "Nettie" Hubbard Bolles, DO [MOM PH1056]

Nettie Bolles (she had married Alden Bolles, who graduated from the ASO in 1898) received her DO degree on 2 March 1894.[62] She has been cited as the first female DO for several reasons. Other than the fact that her name was first alphabetically on the graduation list, Nettie actively taught, published, and practiced osteopathy for her entire life. The other female members of that first graduating class apparently did not continue practicing for more than a few years. After graduating, Nettie Bolles joined the faculty as the instructor of anatomy, filling the position vacated by William Smith and becoming the first female faculty member in the profession.[63] Shortly afterwards, she distinguished herself further as the first editor and publisher of the *Journal of Osteopathy*.[64]

In 1896, Dr. Bolles moved to Colorado, becoming the first practicing osteopath in that state.[65] The next year, she founded a new osteopathic college, which she named the Western Institute of Osteopathy, making her the first woman president of an osteopathic college. Her husband, Alden Bolles, graduated from the ASO in 1898, and a year later they changed the name of their school to the Bolles Institute of Osteopathy.[66] Two years later they again changed the name to the Colorado College of Osteopathy. The school was taken over by the ASO in 1904.[67]

In 1897, Nettie Bolles became the first vice president of the American Association for the Advancement of Osteopathy[68] (later renamed the American Osteopathic Association [AOA]), and in 1898 became the founding president of the Associated Colleges of Osteopathy.[69] For many years, Nettie served with distinction in high-ranking positions in the AOA and in 1917 she became the first woman to be nominated as president of the organization. She was also the first osteopathic physician to serve on the Colorado Board of Medical Examiners. In 1925, the governor of Colorado chose Dr. Bolles to be one of only ten women to represent the state at the International Council on Women in Washington, DC.[70]

Dr. Nettie Bolles was also a founding member of the Osteopathic Women's National Association and served as president three times. She was honored by the osteopathic profession in 1925 with the prestigious AOA Distinguished Service Certificate for "Pioneering in Osteopathy as a Profession for Women."[71]

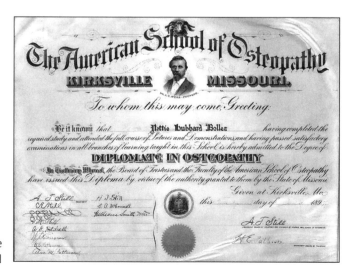

Diploma of Nettie Bolles, the first female Diplomate in Osteopathy. [MOM D290]

Nettie Bolles died on 23 February 1930,[72] but her legacy lived on. Her daughter, Esther Bolles, graduated from the Andrew Taylor Still College of Osteopathy and Surgery in 1924 and was secretary to the Colorado State Board of Examiners in Basic Sciences for thirty-six years. Esther married classmate C. Robert Starks, DO (class of 1925), who was the only person ever to serve two full terms as president of the AOA.[73] Nettie's grandson, C. Robert Starks Jr., also became an osteopathic physician and practiced in Denver for many years.[74]

Mamie Harter, DO

Mamie Bass Harter (Thornburgh), DO (sometimes spelled Thornburg or Thorneburgh) from Sedalia, Missouri, also received her DO degree on 2 March 1894 as part of the first official graduating class from the ASO. The school's records indicate that she had a teacher's certificate before starting her osteopathic studies.[75] She practiced in her hometown of Sedalia in the 1890s, and in Charter Oak, Iowa, between 1904 and 1907.

Her marriage to W. B. Thornburgh was announced in the *Journal of Osteopathy* in July 1902. There is no further information on Dr. Mamie Harter in the osteopathic directories after the year 1907.[76]

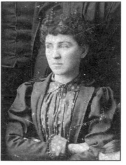

Mamie Harter (Thornburgh), DO
[detail of class picture 1895,
MOM 2000.01.18]

Lou J. Kern (Meitz), DO

Lou Kern (Meitz), DO, was from Springfield, Missouri. She graduated on 2 March 1894, although she does not appear in the 1892 class picture. She returned to the ASO in 1897 for additional classes and was issued a new diploma indicating the additional training.[77]

The early osteopathic directories show her practicing in Springfield, Missouri in 1904 and in Zion City, Illinois in 1907. There are no further listings after 1907.

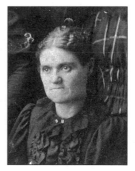

Lou J. Kern, DO
[detail of class picture 1895,
MOM 2000.01.18]

Blanche Still Laughlin, DO

Martha Ellen (Blanche) Still was the youngest child of Andrew Taylor and Mary Elvira Still. In October 1892, at the age of sixteen, Blanche started her studies in osteopathy and was the youngest member of her class. Four of her brothers (Harry, Charlie, Herman, and Fred) were also in the first class. She would have been in the first graduating class had her studies not been interrupted so she could travel to California to care for her brother Fred who had been critically injured in a farm accident.[78] After her brother's death, Blanche returned to Kirksville to continue her education, graduating in 1895.[79]

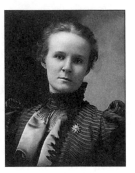

Blanche Still Laughlin, DO
[MOM PH 1614A]

Blanche was a member of the first family of osteopathy and was frequently referred to as the "first lady of osteopathy" for her work serving as the official hostess for osteopathic functions in Kirksville. It was Blanche who would organize meals at the Still home, and she seldom knew how many people to prepare for since her father would invite people to dinner as he met them throughout the day. On any given day, up to eighteen people would show up for the evening meal.[80]

One would be hard pressed to credit anyone else (other than her father) for being more deeply involved in the early years of osteopathy than Dr. Blanche Still. She worked as the secretary and as the triage officer, directing patients to the most appropriate physician; however, there is no evidence that she actively practiced osteopathy.[81]

In 1895, Blanche replaced Nettie Bolles as editor in chief of the *Journal of Osteopathy*, creating the new Women's Page, which was devoted exclusively to women and their relationship to osteopathy. In the first Women's Page, Blanche stated, "This department will consist exclusively of communications from lady Osteopaths, who uphold the science. Osteopathy is today doing more for women than any other science or profession."[82]

In April 1900, Blanche married George M. Laughlin, DO (ASO class of 1900), an orthopedic surgeon who was also a prominent leader of the osteopathic profession during its incipiency. Blanche and George had two children: Mary Jane, born in 1914, and George Andrew, born in 1918.

Many of Blanche's activities were related to the promotion of osteopathy. In the early days, there were so many patients traveling to and staying in Kirksville while receiving care at the osteopathic infirmary and later at the osteopathic hospital, that a group of citizens, including Blanche, organized the Sojourners Club to cater to the nonmedical needs of the patients. The Sojourners Club remains active in Kirksville to this day.[83] It was Blanche Still Laughlin who had the honor of laying the cornerstone of the first permanent osteopathic hospital, the Hospital of the American School of Osteopathy, in 1905.[84]

In her parents' later years, Blanche moved into the Still home to care for her ill mother, who died in 1910, and then again later for her father, who had suffered a minor stroke in 1914 and died on 12 December 1917.[85] Following the death of her father, it was assumed that the presidency of the ASO would go to Blanche's oldest brother, Charles, who was vice president of the ASO and had already taken over the day-to-day operations following their father's stroke. However, through maneuvering of the stock, control of the school was given to George Still, DO, a grandnephew of the founder. Although George Still was a competent administrator and the school continued to thrive under his direction, his appointment as president over Charles caused a split in the Still family. Blanche and her husband sided with her brother Charles and left the school after the takeover.[86]

In 1922, Blanche and George Laughlin founded the A. T. Still College of Osteopathy and Surgery in Kirksville, located just two city blocks from the ASO. A mere month after the competing school opened, George Still, the new president of ASO, was killed in a tragic gun accident. Two years later, in 1924, deprived of the strong leadership of George Still, the board of trustees resigned, the shareholder's stock was placed for sale, and the ASO closed. George Laughlin, assisted by Dr. Harry Still, purchased the ASO's stock and merged the two osteopathic schools.[87] The resulting school continues to function today as the A. T. Still University, Kirksville College of Osteopathic Medicine. Over the front door of the original building of the osteopathic college founded by Blanche and her husband is carved the name A. T. Still College of Osteopathy and Surgery. The building, still a landmark of the A.T. Still University campus, is now dedicated to osteopathic research. Blanche and George Laughlin also founded the Laughlin Osteopathic Hospital in Kirksville and the Laughlin Osteopathic Hospital School of Nursing.

In 1934, Blanche donated historic items that formed the nucleus of the collection at the A. T. Still Memorial Museum. The collection was originally housed in two display cases donated by the Psi Sigma Alpha national honor fraternity and located on the campus of the Kirksville College of Osteopathy and Surgery. This collection has continued to grow and today is the Museum of Osteopathic Medicine.[88] Blanche and George donated their home on South Osteopathy Avenue in Kirksville for the creation of the Community Nursing Home. Blanche also donated 1,150 acres of land for the creation of Thousand Hills State Park located just north of the city.

Blanche lived her entire life in Kirksville and died in 1959 at the age of eighty-three.[89] At the time of her death, the osteopathic profession to which she had dedicated her life was in the early stages of a struggle that was threatening to tear it apart (see pp. 87–92). Blanche was aware that the profession of osteopathic medicine was in mortal danger, but she did not live to see the resolution of that struggle. No doubt Blanche would have been proud to know that the osteopathic profession has not only survived, but has gone on to become the fastest growing segment of American health care.

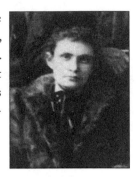

Annie Peters
[detail of class picture 1892/93, MOM 2007.09.01]

Annie Peters

Annie Peters was a member of the inaugural class of the ASO in 1892. There are no records to indicate that she or her husband, Mason Peters (also a member of the ASO inaugural class), ever graduated from the school. The osteopathic directory does, however, list Annie Peters as a practicing osteopath in Kansas City, Missouri, from 1904 to 1910, but not her husband.[90] There are no further entries after that date. It is possible that Annie completed her osteopathic education at one of the other early osteopathic colleges.

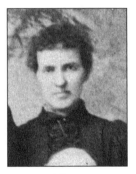

J. Gentry
[detail of class picture 1892/93, MOM 2007.09.01]

J. Gentry

J. Gentry, along with her husband, G. Gentry, were members of the original class of the ASO, however there is no record of either graduating from the school. There is no information as to why the Gentrys did not complete their medical education nor has there been any other information found in the national archives of the osteopathic profession.

Notes

1. A translation of Louis Pasteur's 1857 "Physiological Theory of Fermentation" is available at http://biotech.law.lsu.edu/cphl/history/articles/pasteur.htm#papersII (accessed 22 June 2009).

2. Holmes, "Currents and Counter-Currents in Medical Science," in *Medical Essays, 1842–1882*, 203.

3. Duffy, *The Healers*, 91–97.

4. Armstrong and Armstrong, *Great American Medicine Show*, 1–2.

5. Still, *Autobiography*, 27. On the life of Andrew Taylor Still, see also Trowbridge, *Andrew Taylor Still*; Gevitz, *The DOs*, 1–22; and Adler and Northup, *100 Years of Osteopathic Medicine*, pt. 1.

6. Trowbridge, *Andrew Taylor Still*, 13–19.

7. Still, *Autobiography*, 45, 94; and Laughlin, "Asks if A. T. Still Was Ever a Real Doctor," *Osteopathic Physician* 15, no. 1 (1909): 8.

8. C. E. Still, *Frontier Doctor, Medical Pioneer*, 28–29; and Zornow, *Kansas*, 142.

9. Still, *Autobiography*, 92–94, 224, 326; and Trowbridge, *Andrew Taylor Still*, 89–93.

10. Still, *Autobiography*, 59.

11. Marovia Still Clark, "Reminiscences," 1919, quoted in Trowbridge, *Andrew Taylor Still*, 68.

12. Still, *Autobiography*, 62.

13. C. E. Still, *Frontier Doctor, Medical Pioneer*, 47.

14. C. E. Still, *Frontier Doctor, Medical Pioneer*, 81.

15. Still, *Autobiography*, 98.

16. Still, *Autobiography*, 97–98; Still, "Dr. Still's Department," *Journal of Osteopathy* 6 (Aug. 1899); and Trowbridge, *Andrew Taylor Still*, 94.

17. Still, *Autobiography*, 108.

18. Hildreth, *Lengthening Shadow of Dr. Andrew Taylor Still*, 112.

19. Mayba, *Bonesetters and Others*, 22–27; and Gevitz, *The DOs*, 17–19.

20. Korr et al., *Physiological Basis of Osteopathic Medicine*.

21. Still, *Osteopathy, Research and Practice*, vii.

22. C. E. Still, *Frontier Doctor, Medical Pioneer*, 98–99.

23. DiGiovanna, *Encyclopedia of Osteopathy*, 21.

24. C. E. Still, *Frontier Doctor, Medical Pioneer*, 86–87.

25. C. E. Still, *Frontier Doctor, Medical Pioneer*, 42; Walter, *First School of Osteopathic Medicine*, 1; and Trowbridge, *Andrew Taylor Still*, 120–24.

26. Still, *Autobiography*, 112–13.

27. Gevitz, *The DOs*, 19.

28. Still, *Autobiography*, 113.

29. Walter, *First School of Osteopathic Medicine*, 11, 30.

30. Jackson, "Andrew Taylor Still, MD, DO," *Chiropractic History* 20, no. 2 (Dec. 2000): 15–24.

31. Still, *Autobiography*, 119–23.

32. Still, *Autobiography*, 122, 124.

33. C. E. Still, *Frontier Doctor, Medical Pioneer*, 90–94.

34. Still, *Autobiography*, 112–13, 125; and C. E. Still, *Frontier Doctor, Medical Pioneer*, 95–96.

35. Trowbridge, *Andrew Taylor Still*, 133–34, 137–38.

36. Handbill distributed in Hannibal, MO, announcing his oration and prayer delivered 4 July 1891; original in MOM.

37. Booth, *History of Osteopathy*, 32–34.

38. C. E. Still, *Frontier Doctor, Medical Pioneer*, 98.

39. Harry Still, "Some Early Recollections of My Father in the Discovery and Development of Osteopathy," quoted in Booth, *History of Osteopathy*, 57.

40. Gevitz, *The DOs*, 20.

41. Hildreth, *Lengthening Shadow of Dr. Andrew Taylor Still*, 20–22.

42. Hildreth, *Lengthening Shadow of Dr. Andrew Taylor Still*, 13–15; C. E. Still, *Frontier Doctor, Medical Pioneer*, 101; and Gevitz, *The DOs*, 20.

43. Bunting, "How Osteopathy Got Its First Recognition in Kirksville," *Journal of Osteopathy* 5, no. 10 (March 1899): 473–75.

44. Walter, *First School of Osteopathic Medicine*, 2; and Still, *Autobiography*, 273.

45. Walter, *First School of Osteopathic Medicine*, 47.

46. Smith, "Four Years Ago, Dr. Wm. Smith Gives an Account of His First Visit to Dr. Still." *Journal of Osteopathy* 3 (Sept. 1896): 6; and Smith, "Reviews Pioneer Days," *Osteopathic Physician* 3 (Jan. 1903): 1. See also Still, *Autobiography*, 146–54; and Trowbridge, *Andrew Taylor Still*, 143.

47. Violette, *History of Adair County*, 254–56; Hildreth, *Lengthening Shadow of Dr. Andrew Taylor Still*, 30; and Walter, *First School of Osteopathic Medicine*, 14.

48. Still, *Autobiography*, 162.

49. Still, "Our Platform," *Journal of Osteopathy* 9 (Oct. 1902): 342.

50. Still, *Osteopathy Research and Practice*, vii.

51. Palmer, *The Chiropractor*, 2.

52. American Chiropractic Association, "What is Chiropractic?," accessd 7 July 2010, http://www.acatoday.org/level2_css.cfm?T1ID=13&T2ID=61.

53. A comprehensive search of the archives of the Museum of Osteopathic Medicine/ National Center for Osteopathic History and the American School of Osteopathy shows that a J. Strother was a member of the inaugural class of the ASO, but there is no evidence that he ever completed his studies or received a DO diploma. A student by the name of Strother graduated from the ASO in 1898, after the founding of the first chiropractic school. A close examination of the pictures of these two individuals suggests that they were two different people.

54. Hildreth, *Lengthening Shadow of Dr. Andrew Taylor Still*, 44–45.

55. Gregory, *Spinal Treatment*, xxx.

56. The Edwin Smith Papyrus originated during the reign of Djoser, second pharaoh of the Third Dynasty of the Old Kingdom. The papyrus may have been written by Imhotep, the pharaoh's vizier, architect, and physician. The Edwin Smith Papyrus is currently maintained at the New York Academy of Medicine in New York City.

57. Walter, *First School of Osteopathic Medicine*, 7.

58. Duffy, *The Healers*, 270–77.

59. Hildreth, *Lengthening Shadow of Dr. Andrew Taylor Still*, 112, 412.

60. Walter, *First School of Osteopathic Medicine*, 9–12; and Walter, *Women and Osteopathic Medicine*, 15, 20–21.

61. Trowbridge, *Andrew Taylor Still*, 144; Walter, *Women and Osteopathic Medicine*, 10; and Bolles, "Dr. Still's Regard for Woman's Ability," *JAOA* 17 (Jan. 1918): 250.

62. Walter, *First School of Osteopathic Medicine*, 9.

63. "The First Woman Doctor of Osteopathy," *Forum of Osteopathy* (April 4, 1930): 14.

64. "Mrs. Nettie H. Bolles: Editor and Publisher," *Journal of Osteopathy* 1 (July 1894): 2–3.

65. Walter, *First School of Osteopathic Medicine*, 26.

66. Booth, *History of Osteopathy*, 88–89.

67. Fitzgerald, "Women in History, Pioneers of the Profession," *The DO* 25 (Dec. 1984): 67–71.

68. "Death of Jeanette Hubbard Bolles," *Forum of Osteopathy* 4 (April 1930): 14.

69. Booth, *History of Osteopathy*, 274.

70. Walter, *First School of Osteopathic Medicine*, 181–83.

71. Ibid.

72. "Death of Jeanette Hubbard Bolles," *Forum of Osteopathy* 4 (April 1930): 14.

73. Walter, *First School of Osteopathic Medicine,* 235; and "Dr. and Mrs. Starks," *The DO* 14 (Feb. 1974): 56–57.

74. Correspondence to Larry C. Evans, undated, in Robert Starks Sr., DO, biographical file, MOM/NCOH.

75. ASO, Student Records Box #1, 1892–1898, MOM/NCOH.

76. Cheryl Gracey, "Who Was in the First Class of Osteopathy?" Reference paper, undated, MOM/NCOH.

77. ASO, Student Records Box #1, 1892–1898, MOM/NCOH.

78. Walter, *First School of Osteopathic Medicine,* 18.

79. C. E. Still, *Frontier Doctor, Medical Pioneer,* 155.

80. Hildreth, *Lengthening Shadow of Dr. Andrew Taylor Still,* 44–45.

81. Walter, *First School of Osteopathic Medicine,* 30; and "Dr. Blanche Still Laughlin Dies," *Journal of Osteopathy* 64, no. 12 (Dec. 1959): 48.

82. *Journal of Osteopathy* 1, no. 1 (May 1894): 3; and "Women's Page," *Journal of Osteopathy* 1, no. 9 (Jan. 1895): 4.

83. Still Family Biography File, MOM Archives.

84. "Program at the Missouri Osteopathic Association," *Journal of Osteopathy* 13 (June 1906): 201.

85. Walter, *Women and Osteopathic Medicine,* 11; Trowbridge, *Andrew Taylor Still,* 196; and Walter, *First School of Osteopathic Medicine,* 103.

86. Walter, *First School of Osteopathic Medicine,* 87, 99; and "ASO Owners Split Up: New School Threatened," [Kirksville, MO] *Express,* 18 Jan. 1918, p. 1.

87. Walter, *First School of Osteopathic Medicine,* 111, 130–43, 147–49.

88. "Preserving Heritage, A Retrospective Journey," *Now and Then,* Spring 2005, 1.

89. Walter, *First School of Osteopathic Medicine,* 335.

90. Cheryl Gracey, "Who Was in the First Class of Osteopathy?" Reference Paper, undated, MOM/NOCH.

Chapter Three

The Early Years of Osteopathy, 1895–1929

"There is a profession ... which is peculiarly adapted to women, which is fascinating, satisfactory, and directly beneficial to mankind ... it is Osteopathy."

Jeanette "Nettie" Bolles, DO

"In the early days, women physicians and Osteopathy were both pioneers—and being a pioneer gave call for every bit of persistence, versatility, originality, adaptability, diplomacy, and pugnacity one might possess, because each, in turn, was needed."

Roberta Wimer-Ford, DO

BY THE TIME THE FIRST CLASS GRADUATED IN 1894, the number of students wishing to pursue training in osteopathy easily exceeded the small capacity of the original school building. Likewise, the number of patients also far exceeded the capacity of the available treatment facilities. To accommodate this early explosive growth, Dr. Still purchased sixty-one acres of land just west of the original school property,[1] and on 6 August 1894, A. T. Still's sixty-sixth birthday, ground was broken for a new infirmary building. Dedicated on 10 January 1895, the A. T. Still Infirmary contained seventeen operating (treatment) rooms and lecture halls (the largest of which could hold 250 students), and a dissection room on the third floor.[2]

A reporter for the *Kirksville Graphic* visited the A. T. Still Infirmary in the fall of 1895 and wrote:

The hall and reception rooms were thronged with patients "waiting their turns" for treatment. The greatest rush occurs in the forenoon, and the scene about the Infirmary from early morning until noon beggars description. From over the hills, in every direction, patients can be seen wending their way, some in carriages, others in invalid chairs wheeled by attendants,

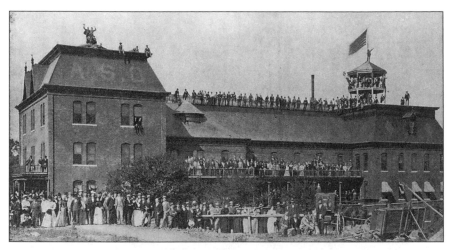

American School of Osteopathy, Infirmary Building with annexes, ca. 1897. [Museum Collection, MOM]

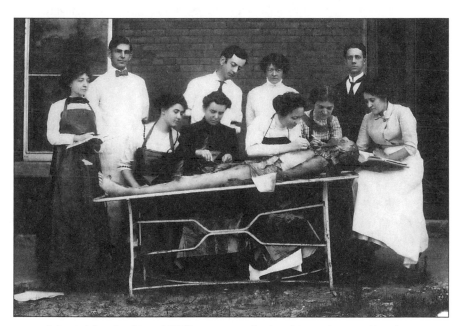

Anatomical dissection class, ca. 1895. There were seven female and three male osteopathic students in the class. [MOM PIC-DIS-14]

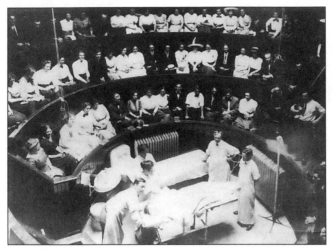

Surgical amphitheatre, often called "The Pit," at the American School of Osteopathy, ca. 1912. Note the number of women in this class. [MOM 2008.75.14]

while many are painfully hobbling along on crutches. There are invalids from almost every corner of the United States, and of every degree of infirmity.... All day long there is a constantly moving stream of humanity going to and from the building, while every train brings in a new detachment of patients.[3]

As word spread of the new infirmary and more people sought out osteopathic treatment, the Wabash Railroad advertised "four daily passenger trains into Kirksville" with special day return fares "for the benefit of patients of the A. T. Still Infirmary."[4] Hotels and other businesses sprang up to serve the four to five hundred patients who were in Kirksville at any given time to receive osteopathic treatments.[5] The A. T. Still Maternity Hospital, which opened in 1894, soon expanded to adapt to the growing need for treatments and surgery and was converted into a surgical sanitarium. When this building became inadequate, Arthur Hildreth, DO, a member of the original class of the American School of Osteopathy (ASO), opened the St. Louis branch of the A. T. Still Infirmary.[6] Some of the success may have been due to Dr. Still's policy that at least one woman DO be on duty at the infirmary at all times to accommodate any woman who preferred to be treated by a female physician.[7]

As the school expanded its physical facilities, it also worked to acquire the most up-to-date and innovative equipment available at the time. Only two years after the first X-ray machine was introduced in the United States, the A. T. Still Infirmary ordered the largest and most modern X-ray machine available. In early

1899, the machine arrived and was installed, only the second X-ray machine in existence west of the Mississippi River.[8]

The ASO was also growing. The class that began in October 1895 had twenty-eight students; a new class began in January 1896 with another twenty-three students, and another class began in May with fifty-one students. By the summer of 1896, the ASO had 102 students enrolled and construction was underway on additions to the building that would accommodate a thousand patients and five hundred students.[9]

The curriculum was also being refined; in 1896, a program consisting of four full terms of six months each (later changed to five months each) was established. By 1900, the ASO had over seven hundred students and eighteen faculty and had added new courses that resulted in a program that differed from typical medical schools only in teaching osteopathic methods in place of the use of drugs.

LICENSING

Some of the changes in curriculum were the result of efforts to have states grant licenses to osteopathic physicians. Under the 1892 business charter for the ASO, the school could grant an MD degree, but Dr. Still chose to grant a DO degree and called the graduates "operators" rather than "doctors." In 1894, the school was rechartered under the law regulating educational and scientific institutions, with article 3 of the charter stating the purpose of the college:

> to improve our present system of surgery, obstetrics, and treatment of diseases generally, and place the same on a more rational and scientific basis, and to impart information to the medical profession, and to grant and confer such honors and degrees as are usually granted and conferred by reputable medical colleges.[10]

During this time, however, state medical associations were struggling to establish licensing laws and licensing boards, efforts that were complicated by the American Medical Association's (AMA's) code of ethics, which prohibited its members from consulting with homeopaths and other irregular doctors. Some states established two licensing boards, one for orthodox doctors and another for homeopaths; New York had a third board for licensing eclectic physicians. Eventually, state medical associations worked with homeopathic and eclectic medical schools to adapt their theories and curriculum so that licensing laws could cover both "regulars" and "irregulars." Ironically, these groups often joined forces to oppose licensing of the newest form of medicine—osteopathy—so that even though the first osteopathic college was in Missouri, Vermont was the first state to license osteopathic physicians in November 1896, followed by North Dakota in February 1897. Finally, on 4 March 1897, osteopathic medicine was legalized in its founding state. When the governor of Missouri signed the osteopathic licensing bill, the whole town of Kirksville erupted into one large celebration.[11] A number of states approved the licensing of osteopathic physicians in the years following, but it was not until 1923 that osteopathic physicians could be fully licensed in most states.

Although orthodox physicians were often opposed to the licensing of osteo-paths, there were many osteopathic patients who were willing to pressure states to adopt licensing laws. One famous example is Mark Twain, who in 1901 testified before the New York legislature on behalf of members of the osteopathic profession who were seeking full licensure there. Twain's interest in osteopathic medicine began in 1896 when he lost his two-year-old daughter to meningitis and became disillusioned with orthodox medicine. When another daughter developed epilepsy, it was natural that Mark Twain would seek alternative treatment. He contacted Dr. Still asking for a good osteopath in New York, where he was living at the time, and was so pleased with the improvement in his daughter's condition while under the care of George Helmer, DO, that he became a devoted supporter of osteopathy.[12]

COMPETITION IN KIRKSVILLE

Only a few years after Dr. Still founded the ASO, additional osteopathic medical colleges opened. In 1897, Marcus Ward, a member of the ASO's first graduating class, opened the Great Columbian School of Osteopathy, Medicine, and Surgery just a short walk from the original school in Kirksville. Ward had originally been a patient of Dr. Still and had become fascinated with osteopathy. He was one of the original shareholders of the ASO and served as vice president of the institution under Dr. Still. After graduating, the new Dr. Ward had a falling out with Dr. Still and left Kirksville in May 1894 to attend the Ohio Medical School of Cincinnati, where he received an MD degree. He returned to Kirksville in April 1897 and started an osteopathic practice, then in November of the same year, with the financial backing of some local Kirksville businessmen, Dr. Ward opened the Great Columbian School of Osteopathy, Medicine, and Surgery, offering a two-year course resulting in a DO degree, with an optional third year so that students could also receive an additional MD degree.[13]

The Great Columbian School, however, held a philosophy that differed significantly from Dr. Still's, teaching and encouraging the use of the full scope of drugs, including the traditional unproven and highly toxic medications rejected by the ASO. The resentment between Dr. Still and Dr. Ward came to a head when Dr. Ward claimed that he was the sole originator of "True Osteopathy," which he defined as a combination of *materia medica*, surgery, and manipulative therapy.[14]

The Great Columbian School was short lived and closed during the fall session of 1900 when Dr. Ward lost his financial backers. The school had only three graduating classes, and the students enrolled in and attending the Great Columbian School at the time classes were suspended were permitted to transfer to the ASO to complete their osteopathic training.[15]

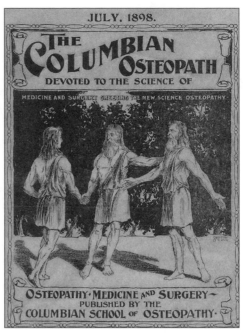

Cover of July 1898 *The Columbian Osteopath*. Dr. Ward's concept of "true osteopathy" was the meeting of the ancient sciences of medicine and surgery with the youthful science of osteopathy. [MOM 1982.643.01]

SPREAD OF OSTEOPATHIC COLLEGES

Additional osteopathic colleges opened in rapid succession. By the turn of the century there were osteopathic medical schools located in the major cities of Los Angeles, Minneapolis, Boston, Philadelphia, San Francisco, Des Moines, Milwaukee, Chicago, Denver, and Buffalo. There were also osteopathic colleges in the smaller cities of Wilkes-Barre, Pennsylvania; Ottawa, Kansas; Franklin, Kentucky; Fargo, North Dakota; Keokuk, Iowa; and Quincy, Illinois.[16] Extracurricular activities were important at the early osteopathic colleges. Students competed in both intramural and intercollegiate sports, and the ASO osteopaths competed in football against much larger universities such as Notre Dame and Texas. Female athletics consisted mostly of swimming, basketball, and tennis, and were an integral part of the athletic program. Other activities were also encouraged, such as bands and glee clubs.

Most of these early osteopathic colleges no longer exist, having closed, merged with, or been bought by other osteopathic colleges. One school, the College of

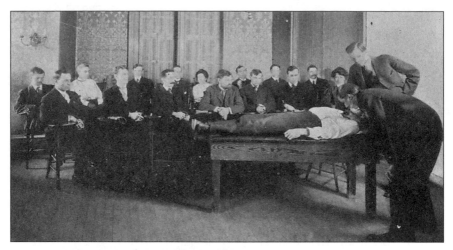

Instruction in physical diagnosis at Philadelphia College and Infirmary of Osteopathy, 1907. [Eighth Annual Announcement, Philadelphia College & Infirmary of Osteopathy session of 1906–1907, Museum Collection, MOM]

Osteopathic Physicians and Surgeons in Los Angeles, was converted to an allopathic medical school in 1961. Only three of the osteopathic colleges that opened before the turn of the last century continue to exist and thrive: A. T. Still University of Health Sciences/Kirksville College of Osteopathic Medicine, founded as the American School of Osteopathy in 1892; Des Moines University, College of Osteopathic Medicine, founded in 1898 as the S.S. Still College of Osteopathy; and Philadelphia College of Osteopathic Medicine, founded as the Philadelphia College and Infirmary of Osteopathy in 1899.

The science of osteopathy was introduced to Great Britain in July 1898 by John Martin Littlejohn, DO, who delivered a lecture on osteopathy to the Society of Science, Letters, and Art in London. Dr. Littlejohn founded the American College of Osteopathic Medicine and Surgery in Chicago in 1900; by 1913 he had left America for London where he established the British School of Osteopathy in 1917. When Littlejohn developed the curriculum for the British School of Osteopathy, he used the outline of coursework developed by the US Associated Colleges of Osteopathy, but excluded *materia medica* and surgery. The British School of Osteopathy had its first graduates in 1925 and remains today a well-respected college of osteopathy. From the British school, osteopathy spread throughout Europe and Australia. The majority of European-trained DOs would be considered osteopaths under the definition of the World Osteopathic Health Organization, meaning that they practice manipulation as a complete and independent diagnostic and therapeu-tic modality, but are not trained in the full spectrum of medicine (there are, however, osteopaths who are also physicians).[17] It is imporant to note that the distinction between an osteopath and an osteopathic physician did not exist in the early years. In fact, although Dr. Still used surgery and some medications, his form of osteo-pathic practice was closer to what international osteopaths practice today than to the broad form of osteopathy, medicine, and surgery practiced today in America, where manipulative therapy has largely become an adjunct to the practice of medi-cine and surgery. Both American-trained osteopathic physicians and international osteopaths are taught the osteopathic philosophy of treating the whole person based on the understanding of the principals of body unity, self-healing, and the interrela-tionship of structure and function.

American Osteopathic Association

In 1897, the profession organized the American Association for the Advancement of Osteopathy (AAAO). Women were instrumental in the AAAO from the very beginning, and the need for a national association became very apparent with the rapid uncontrolled growth of osteopathic colleges. One of the organization's first tasks was to attempt to control the irregular osteopathic colleges.[18] The AAAO set standards for the profession, which included determining the minimum length of study, shaping a uniform curriculum, and setting guidelines for the selection of students and faculty. They also determined the requirements for additional colleges of osteopathy to join the organization.[19] The first organizational meeting took place on 6 February 1897 when students and physicians from the ASO established a

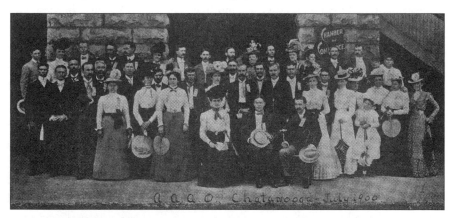

The 1900 convention of the American Association for the Advancement of Osteopathy, held in Chattanooga, Tennessee. [MOM 1976.170.01]

national organization to promote and regulate the profession. They appointed a committee of sixteen students, four from each class. The committee, composed of both male and female students, submitted a constitution on 13 March 1897. A copy of the proposed constitution was sent to the other colleges of osteopathy along with an invitation to attend the first meeting, to be held on 19 April 1897. That meeting was the first annual convention of the AAAO and the first vice president of the association was Nettie Bolles. In 1901, the AAAO changed its name to the American Osteopathic Association (AOA); the annual meeting of the AOA continues today as the largest and most attended medical seminar in the profession. In 1903, the AOA required that for any DO to be accepted as a member, they must have graduated from an osteopathic college that meets the standards of the American Colleges of Osteopathy, which had been founded in 1898, with Nettie Bolles as its first president, to regulate the educational processes of the osteopathic colleges.[20]

RAPID UNCONTROLLED EXPANSION

In the early years of osteopathy, the profession grew rapidly, but this expansion was largely uncontrolled. This unrestrained growth was the result of the extraordinarily lax or in some instances, nonexistent laws of the time. Virtually anyone who wanted to open a medical school, DO or MD, could do so with minimal requirements.[21] From the late nineteenth century through the early years of the twentieth century, a multitude of osteopathic medical schools opened. There were even correspondence schools that granted DO degrees through home study. Most of these schools did not meet the requirements of the AOA, but in the early years AOA approval was not legally needed for a school to exist and to confer the DO degree. In these formative years, mostly as the result of lobbying by the AMA, many states would not grant unlimited medical licenses to osteopathic physicians, and those states that did required graduation from an approved school.[22]

In 1902 the AOA mandated that all approved colleges of osteopathic medicine must extend the course of instruction to three years of nine months each, but it was not until 1905 that all of the approved schools were in full compliance.[23] Osteopathic medical schools not approved by the AOA, however, could not be made to improve their educational standards. This situation was not unique to osteopathy; at that time, there were many allopathic, homeopathic, and eclectic medical colleges that did not meet the educational requirements of their respective national regulatory bodies.

In many states, the difficulty in obtaining full and unlimited medical licenses for osteopathic physicians was due partly to the lack of control over the quality of education provided by the nonapproved and unregulated osteopathic schools, but a significant part of the opposition came from organized medicine. The AMA would first begin its opposition by resisting full medical licensure for DOs. After being successful it would next initiate direct legal action against individual osteopathic physicians for practicing medicine without a license.[24] Despite opposition by the AMA, by 1913 thirty-nine states had passed some kind of law for the licensing of osteopathic practitioners, and by 1923 this number had risen to forty-six states.[25]

The MD-granting schools of the time, however, were just as chaotic and in some respects even more so. The allopathic, homeopathic, physiomedical, and eclectic medical schools all conferred the MD degree on their graduates, with the result being that the general public often did not understand what qualifications their physician actually had. Dr. A. T. Still chose to bestow the DO degree to the graduates of the osteopathic colleges with the intention of distinguishing them from the myriad of other medical practitioners of the time.[26]

The first osteopathic physician permitted to testify in a court of law was Florence McCoy, DO, who in May 1902 testified concerning a patient who had been injured while getting off a streetcar in Toledo, Ohio. The attorney for the streetcar company objected to her testimony, alleging that because Dr. McCoy was an osteopathic physician, she was not licensed to practice medicine. Dr. McCoy pointed out that the Ohio legislature had just three weeks previously passed a law allowing the licensing of osteopathic physicians in Ohio, and therefore she was permitted to testify. The *Toledo Times* reported that the judge "allowed Dr. McCoy, a lady osteopath, to give testimony, thus placing osteopathic medicine on an equal basis with other departments of medical science, as far as the courts were concerned."[27]

In 1903, the AOA encouraged the entire profession to change much of the outdated terminology used in early osteopathy

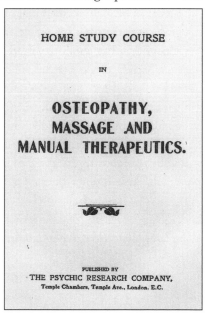

Inside cover of a correspondence course in osteopathy, ca. 1900.
[MOM WB940.H765 1902]

that the organization felt trivialized the profession. The DO degree, which stood for "diplomate in osteopathy," was to be changed to "doctor of osteopathy." The DO, rather than being referred to as an "operator," should be called a "doctor" or "physician." Instead of the phrase "handling the patient," the DO's activity should be described as "treating the patient." The profession should be referred to as a "practice" rather than a "business" or "work." Finally and most importantly, the term "osteopath" or "osteopathist" was to be changed to "osteopathic physician" to more accurately reflect the medical education and scope of practice for the profession.[28]

A later change was specifically directed at female osteopathic physicians, who were traditionally referred to as "Mrs." or "Miss," while male osteopathic physicians were called "doctor." In 1907, Alice Patterson, DO, published an article in the *Journal of Osteopathy*, insisting that female DOs should be given the same respect as their male counterparts: "They should be called by their professional title and not referred to by their gender."[29]

Ten-Fingered vs. Three-Fingered Osteopaths

In the early years of osteopathy, there was a fundamental conflict over the scope of practice and the range of treatments that should be used. Much of the debate was focused on disagreements between the so-called lesion osteopaths and the broad osteopaths over the inclusion of medications, vaccines, and other medical modalities. The lesion osteopaths were frequently referred to as ten-fingered osteopaths, referring to the full use of both hands to perform osteopathic manipulative therapy. These osteopaths held the most conservative stance on osteopathic philosophy and considered Dr. Still's system to consist of structural diagnosis and manipulative therapy with only minimal use of medicine and surgery.

The broad osteopaths were frequently referred to as three-fingered osteopaths, in reference to the three fingers needed to use a hypodermic needle and to write a prescription. These DOs felt that the profession should embrace medications, surgery, and all proven therapeutic modalities available in addition to manipulative therapy. The broad osteopaths envisioned osteopathic physicians as complete physicians competent to treat their patients with all scientifically proven treatments available.

Some of the schools offering primarily manipulative therapy considered themselves to teach pure osteopathy, whereas others were nothing more than diploma mills, operating strictly for the money they could obtain from tuition or from the outright selling of diplomas. The diploma mills were not unique to osteopathic medicine, but were pervasive across all medical education in the United States during that era.

The two groups struggled for the support of the majority of osteopathic physicians, with neither group gaining the upper hand until the 1918/19 influenza pandemic temporarily swung the pendulum toward the side of the lesion osteopaths. At the time, there were no known medications or vaccines available that were effective against this virulent form of influenza virus.[30] MDs found limited success in treating this rapid-spreading pandemic with traditional methods. The DOs however, focused on treatment of the whole person and included hygiene, fluid intake, isolation, and manipulative therapy, and had marked success against the virus with minimal use of medications, for which they received national publicity. The manipulative therapy released disease-fighting white blood cells (lymphocytes) into the circulatory system to bolster the patient's immune system and reduce the build-up of fluids that frequently led to pneumonia as an often-fatal aftereffect of influenza. This was a major victory for the ten-fingered (lesion) osteopaths, ironically, because many satisfied patients began to rely on a DO as their family doctor. However, the three-fingered (broad) osteopaths soon regained the upper hand. The number of broad osteopaths continued to grow and the movement toward the full integration of all scientifically proven therapies, including the full acceptance of all medications into the osteopathic armamentartium, would prevail.[31]

In 1927, the AOA met with representatives of the Associated Colleges of Osteopathy and the two groups mandated that every approved osteopathic college must teach comparative therapeutics,[32] including medical, biological, and chemical agents, with the intention that the profession be unified in teaching the complete and unlimited scope of medical practice. Previously, all approved osteopathic colleges had taught the use of medications, but some to a greater degree than others. This joint ruling both standardized the training and guaranteed educational standards at least equal to the allopathic medical schools. This mandate was met with enthusiasm by some and criticism by others, both from within and outside of the profession. So two years later, the AOA clarified its policy and initiated a course on supplemental therapeutics, in which it again mandated complete training in the use of biological and chemical agents. To ensure that there would be no further misunderstandings that it intended to include the complete and unlimited scope of medical practice, the AOA added the term "pharmacology" to the subheading of the course title.[33] The official policy of the AOA from 1927 onward was that all osteopathic medical schools in the United States would teach the complete and unlimited scope of practice. The AOA reinforced this requirement in 1929 and has never wavered in its commitment since that time.

Reform of Medical Education

The early debates within the osteopathic profession over the merits of various forms of treatment soon shifted to efforts to improve the educational system and the training of osteopathic physicians. In the early twentieth century, the AMA also worked to raise the level of medical education at member schools. Licensing boards were concerned over the vast differences in the quality of medical education received at different institutions, and were especially concerned about lax standards at medical schools not associated with a college or university. These so-called proprietary institutions often had few if any entrance requirements and courses were often taught by practitioners who had trained through an apprentice system rather than in an academic environment. The AMA attempted to set standards for its member schools, and in 1907, the association's Council on Medical Education asked the Carnegie Foundation for the Advancement of Teaching to investigate the state of medical education.

In 1909, the Carnegie Foundation, with the cooperation of the US Congress and in cooperation with the AMA's Council on Medical Education, appointed a commission headed by Abraham Flexner, a graduate of Johns Hopkins University. Over the next year, Flexner conducted an extensive study of medical education in the United States and Canada, visiting a total of 155 schools, including 123 allopathic, 15 homeopathic, 8 eclectic, 1 physiomedical, and 8 osteopathic medical schools.[34] At that time, the state of medical education was little more than a mockery. At the majority of medical schools, the most important requirement for admission was the student's ability to pay the tuition. Fewer than 25 percent of the medical schools required a secondary school education. The lesser schools would admit even barely literate students, so long as they could afford tuition. Many schools gave no examinations and the students were almost never graded on their abilities. Most of the instruction was in the form of lectures to large groups of students, who rarely had any direct contact with the instructor. In many schools, laboratory training was minimal or nonexistent and the physical facilities were described as decrepit and disgraceful. Hands-on medical experience was frequently scant and sometimes nonexistent. School catalogues often exaggerated the physical facilities and deliberately distorted the school's capabilities.[35]

The effect of Flexner's report, *Medical Education in the United States and Canada* (commonly called the *Flexner Report*), which was released in 1910, was felt throughout all levels of medical education. The report was critical of the majority of the schools Flexner visited, revealing the disorganized and substandard state of medical education and the obvious need for reform of the entire medical educational system.[36] Flexner criticized the osteopathic medical schools (which relied primarily on tuition to cover operating expenses) for their lack of outside funding, which resulted in substandard facilities and equipment. In his report, Flexner stated that the eight osteopathic medical schools, all of which were proprietary institutions, "reek with commercialism."[37] The osteopathic colleges received particular criticism for the few and small osteopathic hospitals available to the young profession.[38] Because DOs were denied admission to MD hospitals, the osteopathic profession was forced to develop its own hospital system with limited resources, and the osteopathic hospital system was still in the early stages of development. The first true full-service osteopathic hospital had only begun operations in 1906, a mere three years before the Flexner inspection. Built by the ASO, it could accommodate fifty to seventy-five patients and had full surgical and obstetrical units.[39]

As a result of Flexner's scathing report, many medical schools closed or merged with other schools. Institutions with the foresight to see that Flexner's report was the beginning of a major reform in medical education searched for ways to upgrade their physical facilities, educational processes, and the quality and quantity of their faculty.[40] All medical schools tightened the requirements for graduation and made them more stringent. In 1910, the Philadelphia College and Infirmary of Osteopathy adopted a four-year curriculum[41] and by 1916 all other approved osteopathic medical schools also adopted a full four-year curriculum.[42] By 1924, all of the unapproved osteopathic schools had either closed or merged with an approved school, and the AOA became the sole accreditation agency for the DO degree. Without this accreditation the unapproved schools could no longer grant DO degrees and they ceased to exist.[43] From the founding of the first osteopathic college in 1892 until 1974, the profession never had more than eight approved colleges.[44]

During this time of reform in medical education, there were also changes in women's access to it. There was a dramatic increase in the numbers of female physicians during the last decades of the nineteenth century, due primarily to an increase in female medical colleges during that period. Between 1850 and 1895, nineteen all-female medical schools had opened. After the ASO and Johns Hopkins began accepting women and other medical schools gradually opened their doors to women, the number of all-female schools decreased, and by 1904, only three remained.[45] Since many coeducational medical schools accepted only

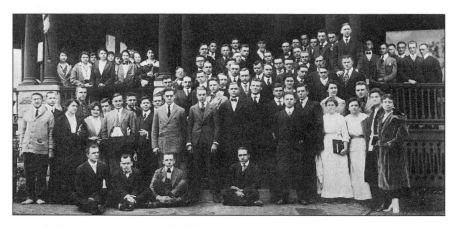

Freshman class of the American School of Osteopathy, 1916/17. This was the last class picture with A. T. Still (center back). [1918 *Osteoblast*, MOM]

a token number of female students, the closing of most of the all-female schools contributed to the sharp decline of female physicians.

Flexner found that in 1909, the number of all-male medical schools that were accepting women was slowly increasing, however, the number of women attending these schools was decreasing. Flexner attributed this decline in female enrollment to a lack of "any strong demand for women physicians," a lack of "any strong ungratified desire on the part of women to enter the profession," or "perhaps both."[46] Flexner also reviewed the failure rates of physicians from 1901 through 1903 and found that students at the all-female medical schools had a failure rate of 4.9 percent whereas the failure rate at the predominately male medical schools was 16.3 percent.[47]

During World War I, there was a temporary surge of female DO and MD medical students due to the drain of male students for the war effort. In 1923, 50 percent of all osteopathic medical students were women, but by 1928 that number had dropped to 12 percent.[48] Around this same time, female osteopathic physicians were organizing their own professional association. At the 1914 AOA Convention held in Philadelphia, the Board of Trustees created a Women's Bureau of Public Health, which was reorganized in 1920 as the Osteopathic Women's National Association. In 1922, the first group of Osteopathic Women's Auxiliaries was organized for the specific purpose of financing and supporting an osteopathic clinic. In short time, auxiliaries were quickly organizing throughout the country. Eventually the auxiliaries grew to a point that it was necessary to appoint a leader. In 1928, Dr. Elizabeth Broach of Atlanta became the national chairperson.[49]

In that same year, the *Forum of Osteopathy* published a plea for additional women to apply to osteopathic medical schools and appealed to female osteopathic physicians to recruit female applicants, imploring that "If osteopathy is a science that as the Old Doctor said, 'opened the door for women' are we women carrying on the work he started for us?"[50] Despite efforts to recruit women, female graduates of osteopathic medical schools still had to overcome the reluctance of the American public to accept female physicians. This was an impediment that all female physicians, DOs and MDs alike, had to face.

WOMEN OF THE EARLY YEARS, BETWEEN 1895 AND 1929

Even when a woman managed to overcome all of the impediments to gaining entrance into a medical school and then triumphed over the chauvinism of her classmates and professors to gain her medical degree, she still found herself treated as a second-rate physician. Female physicians could seldom obtain hospital privileges or faculty positions, and many patients looked upon them with skepticism. A woman's medical practice would struggle to grow, while a man's would flourish. A female physician's femininity was frequently questioned, often by the men who were reluctant to accept any female incursion into a male-controlled profession.

Alice Patterson, DO

Alice Patterson (born Alice Mary Smith) had first been exposed to osteopathy as a child, when Dr. A. T. Still was her family doctor. Alice's mother was one of Dr. Still's early patients when he first moved to Kirksville. He had treated her mother for asthma, and Alice remembered her family being "all but ostracized" by the neighbors because they were patients of the strange Dr. Still.[51]

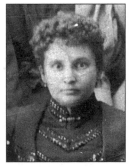

Alice Patterson, DO
[detail of class picture, 1895, MOM 2000.01.18]

After graduating from high school and attending Northeast Missouri State Normal School, Alice Mary Smith married Henry Edorus Patterson, a local businessman, in 1886. In 1893, Alice Patterson and her husband enrolled in the second class of the ASO and graduated in 1895.[52] While still a student, Alice Patterson discovered an osteopathic treatment for gallstones. After graduating, Dr. Patterson joined the ASO faculty as an instructor in obstetrics and gynecology, and clinical instructor. She was also the first assistant in the maternity hospital, providing a regular course of lectures for the ASO on osteopathic obstetrics and diseases of women.[53] Her husband became Dr. Still's secretary and business manager, as well as serving as secretary of the ASO.

Alice Patterson held the title of "chief lady operator" at the A. T. Still Infirmary and became the head of the Department of Obstetrics and Gynecology.[54] In 1900 she became the first vice president of the AAAO.[55]

Helen Barber, DO

Helen Barber graduated from the ASO in 1895. She and her husband, Elmer Barber (also an 1895 graduate of the ASO), founded the National School of Osteopathy (NSO) in Kansas City, Missouri. Almost immediately, animosity developed between the Drs. Barber and their school, and A. T. Still and the ASO—and with good reason. The NSO was nothing more than a diploma mill. The duration of study was much shorter than at the ASO and there were rumors that a diploma could be purchased for a price.[56] In addition, Elmer Barber published two books that he claimed were sufficient to teach anyone the practice of manipulation.

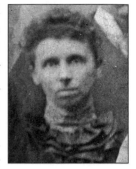

Helen Barber, DO
[detail of class picture, 1895, MOM 2000.02.18]

Hearing the rumors, Dr. Still sent William Smith to meet with the Barbers in Kansas City. Dr. Smith had taught anatomy at the ASO before the Barbers were students, so they had never met him. Using an assumed name, Dr. Smith met with Dr. Elmer Barber, who sold him a DO diploma for $150. Dr. Smith went directly to the Missouri attorney general and filed a complaint against the Barbers and the NSO. The court found that the Barbers were not complying with a state law regarding the length of instruction required before awarding a degree. They were ordered to pay a fine, but the judge did not revoke their charter, determining that the fact that Dr. Smith had already possessed both MD and DO degrees mitigated the charges against them.[57]

When the *Journal of Osteopathy* published an item accusing the Barbers of running a diploma mill, they sued the ASO for libel. After losing the lawsuit in 1900, the Barbers closed the NSO.[58] During the time the school was operational, the NSO issued over fifty DO diplomas. Two of their graduates went on to open diploma mills of their own: the Payne's College of Osteopathy and Optics in Ottawa, Kansas, and the Noe's College of Osteopathy in San Francisco.[59] Since the laws governing medical and osteopathic education during the late nineteenth and early twentieth centuries were extremely lax, there was little legitimate medical educators could do to control unauthorized and substandard schools.

Ada A. Achorn, DO

Ada A. Achorn graduated from the Northern Institute of Osteopathy in Minneapolis in 1896. She was married to classmate Clinton Edwin Achorn, a 1897 graduate, and they moved to Boston where they became the first osteopathic physicians to practice in the state.[60] Dr. Ada Achorn also served as second vice president of the AOA in 1907 and 1908.

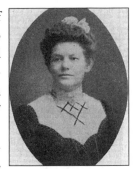

Ada Achorn, DO
[1904 *Osteopathic Physician*, MOM]

In 1897, the Drs. Achorn founded the Boston Institute of Osteopathy, the first osteopathic college on the East Coast. Ada served as secretary of the college with her husband serving as the president. The college changed its name in 1903 to the Massachusetts College of Osteopathy and continued to function as a high-quality osteopathic college until World War II, when so many students and professors were called to serve their country that the school could no longer function. A victim of decreased enrollment and insufficient funding, the Massachusetts College of Osteopathy was forced to close its doors in 1944, a major loss for the profession.

Ella D. Still, DO

Ella Dougherty graduated from the ASO in 1897. After graduation she became a regular operator at the A. T. Still Infirmary and worked closely with Dr. Andrew T. Still. Ella married Summerfield S. Still, who had received his DO degree in 1896 and was the son of Andrew T. Still's older brother James Moore Still. In 1897, when the AAAO was founded, Ella was elected as one of the original trustees. In 1902, Ella served as second vice president, and in 1909 she was elected as first vice president of the AOA.[61]

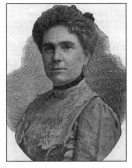

Ella D. Still, DO
[1902 *Osteopathic Physician*, MOM]

In 1898, Ella and her husband founded the S. S. Still College of Osteopathy in Des Moines, Iowa. In 1905, the school consolidated with the ASO. It was closed in June 1905 until a group of professors from the college raised enough money to purchase the school building and reopen it in time for the fall semester. After several more name changes, the school exists today as the University of Des Moines, College of Osteopathic Medicine. Drs. Ella and S. S. Still are still recognized as the founders.[62]

Dr. Ella Still and her husband returned to the ASO in 1913 Ella became the head of the Department of Obstetrics and Gynecology and her husband taught anatomy. George Still, son of Ella and S. S. Still, was also a major figure in the history of osteopathy. George was chief of staff and chief of surgery of the ASO Hospital and later president of the ASO.[63]

Minnie F. Potter, DO, and Cornelia A. Walker, DO

Minnie F. Potter graduated from the ASO in 1898. While still a student, Minnie participated in the founding of the AAAO. Forty years later, Minnie wrote to a former classmate, T. L. Ray, reminiscing about the day they had helped to organize the AOA.

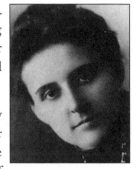

Minnie Potter, DO
[MOM PH-85]

> I know that after our little bunch accepted Aunty Walker's name for "our baby," we began adding to our number as rapidly as we could. If I am correct, there are only four of us left who were the original pioneers of this organization's movement who made their dreams come true. I suppose you remember the picnic supper our class had, down on the green, the afternoon we organized the AOA?[64]

"Our baby" was the AOA and "Aunty Walker" was Cornelia A. Walker, the student who suggested the original name for the organization. Walker graduated in 1898.

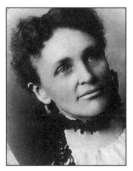

Cornelia A. Walker, DO
(Auntie Walker)
[MOM PH-85]

Carry Nation, DO?

Carry Nation, famous temperance agitator, may have also been an osteopathic physician. She was born in Kentucky in 1846 and her family moved several times before settling in Belton County, Missouri, near Kansas City. Her first husband, Dr. Charles Gloyd, was a physician, but he was also a drunkard who was not able to make a living. The marriage was unsuccessful and the couple soon separated. Gloyd died from the effects of alcoholism shortly after Carry left him. In 1874, Carry married David Nation, a lawyer, minister, and editor who was nineteen years her senior. The couple lived in Texas for a number of years, then moved to Medicine Lodge, Kansas, in 1890 when David became pastor of the Christian Church in nearby Holton and Carry ran a hotel.

On February 28, 1900, while living in Medicine Lodge, Carry noted in her diary that she was studying osteopathy. According to Fran Grace's biography of Nation, some of Carry's acquaintances later speculated that she had earned so much money as an osteopath that she could retire after five years and "devote the remainder of her life to joint smashing."[65]

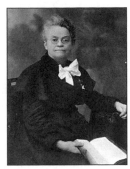
Carry Nation, DO?.
[Kansas State Historical Society]

Carry Nation placed her faith in the natural action of the body to heal itself. In a letter to the editor of the *Barber County Index* in 1900, she wrote "…osteopathy is an intelligent use of the laws of nature removing hindrances and opening up the way for nature to affect her own course."[66] Carry Nation was quite accurately expressing the teachings of A.T. Still, so it seems plausible that she had studied osteopathy, at least informally.

Exhaustive searches of records of the ASO at the National Center for Osteopathic History and the Museum of Osteopathic Medicine reveal no evidence of Carry Nation being enrolled as a student at that institution. There were however, multiple approved and nonapproved osteopathic colleges between 1892 and 1900 and even Elmer Barber's books that claimed to teach all one needed to know to become an osteopath. Because very few of the records remain from the early osteopathic colleges that closed or merged with other schools, it is not possible to document whether Nation attended classes at any of those schools. It does seem, however, that Nation practiced osteopathic medicine and was considered an osteopath in her community. A news item in the *Barber County* (KS) *Index* reported that Carry Nation, DO, had delivered a son for Mr. and Mrs. Ed Tombs on 16 May 1900.

There is evidence that Dr. A.T. Still met with Carry Nation, but that was years after Carry would have received her osteopathic training. The Museum of Osteopathic Medicine has a copy of Nation's autobiography, *The Use and Need of the Life of Carry A. Nation*, published in 1908. On the inside leaf, one of the Still children wrote, "Carry Nation gave this book to Pa when she was here on a lecture tour."[67]

Gene G. Banker, DO
Gene G. Banker was the first female graduate of the Philadelphia College and Infirmary of Osteopathy in 1900, and one of only two students enrolled in the first class. Dr. Banker practiced osteopathic medicine for over sixty years in the Germantown section of Philadelphia until she died at age ninety-nine. She was a beloved general

practitioner and in spite of her small physical stature, became a colossal figure for osteopathic medicine, well known for her osteopathic treatments.[68]

A letter from a grateful patient, Mrs. Marion W. Jenks, written in 1969 at the time of Dr. Banker's death states, "Dr. Banker brought to her practice a cheery optimism: faith, humor, and a zest for living that sustained her to the end. She was very little more than five feet tall, thin of face, with lovely graying hair. But she was wiry, and with strong fingers and wrists she administered treatments. She never became wealthy, because her services were frequently contributed when patients couldn't pay. She was an old fashioned, but wonderful family physician."[69]

Edythe F. Ashmore, DO

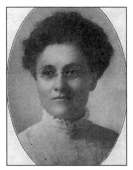

Edythe F. Ashmore, DO
[1916 *Osteopathic Physician,* MOM]

Edythe Ashmore was a 1901 graduate of the S. S. Still College of Osteopathy in Des Moines, Iowa. While practicing osteopathic medicine in Detroit, Dr. Ashmore served as the secretary and treasurer of the Detroit Osteopathic Society and was a member of the Michigan State Board of Examination and Registration in Osteopathy until 1911. She later moved to Los Angles to study at the Los Angeles College of Osteopathy, where she also practiced and was involved in research.[70]

Dr. Ashmore was active in teaching and presented many lectures throughout the country to osteopathic groups and at AOA Conventions. She was a well-known osteopathic lecturer and wrote on a wide variety of subjects including osteopathic manipulative treatment techniques, nervous disorders, osteopathic mechanics, osteopathic nomenclature, spinal lesions, the treatment of neurasthenia, and a variety of other subjects. In addition to her practice, research, writing, and lecturing, Dr. Ashmore was also active in medical politics. At the annual AOA meetings in 1906 and again in 1911, she was elected first vice president of the association. In 1914, Dr. Ashmore left Los Angeles to become head of the Department of Osteopathic Techniques at the ASO where she worked with Dr. A. T. Still. In August of that same year, *The Journal of Osteopathy* announced that Dr. Ashmore was to be the new editor.[71]

Dr. Ashmore also wrote one of the earliest textbooks published on osteopathic manipulative therapy. In 1915, she published *Osteopathic Mechanics,* and in a book review that appeared in *The Journal of Osteopathy,* the reviewer called her book "a real advance in osteopathic teaching." *The Osteopathic Physician* wrote that

Ashmore's book was "the most important thing that has happened to the osteopathic profession in ten years, bar nothing."[72]

Emily Bronson Conger, DO

Emily Bronson Conger became interested in osteopathic medicine after Dr. A. T. Still treated her husband, Anthony Conger, for a stroke in 1895. Colonel Conger (he had been in the Civil War) was chairman of the Republican National Committee, through which he was acquainted with US Senator and Mrs. Joseph P. Foraker from Ohio. The Forakers' son was under treatment at the ASO and Infirmary in Kirksville, Missouri, and the Forakers were so pleased with the care their son was receiving and the excellent progress he was making that they recommended that Col. Conger go to Kirksville for osteopathic treatment.[73]

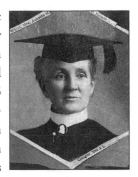

Emily Conger, DO
[MOM PH-86]

In 1895, the colonel spent several months receiving treatment at the infirmary and Mrs. Conger was so impressed with the improvement in her husband's condition that she enrolled in the ASO in 1899, shortly before her husband's death from an unrelated illness. She later became vice president of the AOA.

Emily Conger, along with one of her sons, traveled to the Philippines to work with the American soldiers. While in the Philippines, she also provided medical care for Filipino women and their children, who referred to her as Senora Blanca. She later wrote a book entitled, *An Ohio Woman in the Philippines* that was based on her encounters with the Philippine people.[74]

Florence MacGeorge, DO

Florence MacGeorge graduated from the ASO in 1900. She was born in Tasmania and practiced in New Zealand. Although she lectured throughout the world on the science of osteopathy (she was fluent in French, Italian, and German), the most interesting part of Dr. MacGeorge's story is about how she first became interested in osteopathy.

As a young woman, Florence suffered from failing eyesight accompanied by extreme pain. She traveled far and wide seeking treatment for her worsening eye problems, and

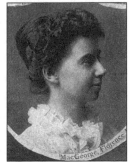

Florence MacGeorge, DO
[MOM PH 420(4)4]

multiple specialists prescribed progressively stronger lenses. She was advised that she use her eyes for only ten to thirty minutes a day, and was confined to a darkened room for the remainder of the time. Florence even consulted with the world-renowned oculist who was Queen Victoria's physician. He took away her glasses and prescribed stinging eye drops, which she used faithfully but received no relief. Eventually she was told that nothing could be done for her failing eyesight and excruciating pain.

Sometime in the 1890s she came across information about Dr. Still and osteopathy and against the advice of her friends who "heard much but knew little" about osteopathy, in an act of desperation, she decided to visit Dr. Still, even though he was a small-town country doctor who did not specialize in eyes.

On her first visit to the osteopathic infirmary, she was told that her problem had nothing to do with her eyes but that her pain and failing vision were the result of an injury to her neck. She was told that her first cervical vertebra (atlas) was twisted, carrying with it the second cervical vertebra (axis), and that the vertebrae were impinging certain fibers of the nervous system. Although there was no trauma immediately associated with her condition, Florence remembered a childhood fall when her sister had attempted to carry her down the stairs. Her sister had cut her forehead in the fall, but Florence was thought to be unharmed.

Florence's first osteopathic treatment adjusted her atlas and axis, returning them to their appropriate positions. This treatment relieved the impingement on the nerves and restored the proper circulation. Her pain was immediately improved and she was assured that there would be no further loss of vision; however because of the length of time since her injury, it was uncertain whether her lost vision would return. She was advised that it would take at least one month to determine if the lost vision could be restored, and that if the vision started to return, she should receive additional treatments until she achieved optimum restoration of vision. Over several months Florence's vision was completely restored.

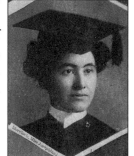

Florence was so impressed with this new science of osteopathy that she applied to and was accepted into the ASO. She kept her enthusiasm for osteopathy throughout her life and did much to spread the word of osteopathy throughout the world.[75]

Josephine Morelock, DO

In 1927, Dr. Josephine Morelock (ASO, 1903) was chosen as the most prominent professional woman in

Josephine Morelock, DO
[MOM PH 86]

Hawaii. It was already unusual for this award to be given to a physician, and this was the first time it had ever been presented to an osteopathic physician.

Dr. Josephine Morelock and her sister Isabelle Morelock, DO, are the osteopathic pioneers of Hawaii. They brought osteopathy to the Hawaiian Islands in 1917. During their ten years in Hawaii, Josephine and Isabelle were responsible for obtaining legislation granting osteopathic physicians the right to practice in Hawaii and creating an independent Board of Osteopathic Examiners. Their work contributed to the high esteem of the osteopathic profession.[76] Each year, A. T. Still University, Kirksville College of Osteopathic Medicine awards the Josephine and Isabelle Morehead Student Scholarship for academic excellence to a worthy student at the university.

Lillie M. Murray, DO, and Anna A. Domann, DO: Blind Osteopaths

The osteopathic profession was ahead of its time not only in freely accepting women into osteopathic medicine, but also in openly considering admission of persons with handicaps. In fact the ASO had two blind students in the class of 1899; however, the names and gender of these students are not recorded.[77]

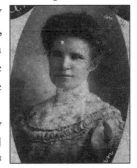

In February 1905, Lillie M. Murray, who was totally blind, received her DO degree from the Southern School of Osteopathy and eventually ran a practice in Tennessee.[78] In June 1905, Anna Domann, who was also totally blind, received her DO degree from the ASO.[79] She later married and became Dr. Anna A. Anderson.

Anna A. Domann, DO
[MOM PH 267(2)2]

Zeo Zoe Wilkins, DO

The sweet-faced girl who posed for her class picture at the ASO in 1905 is probably the most infamous osteopath of all time.[80] Zeo Wilkins was born on a farm in Ohio in the 1880s, the youngest of thirteen children, and grew up in poverty. Besides being beautiful and clever, Zeo had a talent for distorting the truth to her advantage, so many details of her life are sketchy. By 1900, the family had split up and Zeo was living in Cleveland with several of her siblings. While Zeo attended school, her brother Charles worked as a machinist and her sister Irene worked at a

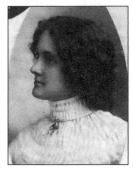

Zeo Zoe Wilkins, DO,
"Osteopathic Femme Fatale"
[MOM PH 267(2)2]

homeopathic college, where she heard about opportunities for women in medicine. Zeo's sister Gertrude completed high school and business college, and earned a teacher's certificate. When Gertrude decided to pursue a medical career, Zeo decided she would also pursue a career in osteopathy, but her motivation was to place herself in a position to meet wealthy men. She and Gertrude chose the ASO, which advertised "women are admitted on the same terms as men." To get around the admissions requirements, Zeo gave her age as nineteen, although she was probably no more than seventeen, and used a copy of her sister's teaching certificate with her own name forged on it. Determined to be successful, Zeo applied herself to her studies and did well in school, but medical studies were not all that occupied her thoughts. Richard Dryer, a classmate and son of a wealthy and prominent banker, caught her fancy. She told a friend she intended to marry him: "I shall get enough money to finance my start in osteopathy and then divorce him."[81]

The details are not clear, but apparently only weeks into the term, the couple eloped. Once her new husband had given her a large amount of money, Zeo filed for divorce and returned to Kirksville to continue her osteopathic studies. Her former husband, despondent over the divorce, may have threatened suicide, or even succeeded; in any case, he did not return to medical school. Zeo, on the other hand, continued to do well in her studies and soon set her sights on Charles Kittredge Garring, a thirty-six-year-old former businessman in his last year of study. Garring was attracted to Zeo not only for her great beauty, but also for her intellectual brilliance. He fell madly in love and they married shortly after his graduation in 1904. The newly minted Dr. Garring set up a practice in an oil rush town in the Indian Territory; meanwhile, Zeo paid her tuition and returned to school in the fall while her husband wrote letters pressuring her to abandon her studies and join him. After she graduated in 1905, Zeo did join her husband and they practiced medicine together, but she was soon distracted by the more appealing of her many male patients.[82]

Apparently Zeo grew tired of her husband—and attracted to his generous life insurance policy. One evening when he arrived home, she shot him at point blank range—twice—claiming later that she thought he was a burglar. The police accepted her explanation and no charges were filed. Her husband, once he recovered from his wounds, filed for divorce and in November 1905 he put up his practice for sale. If he had known about his wife's lovers, he was gentleman enough not to file for divorce on the grounds of infidelity. Dr. Wilkins was now divorced for the second time, but she had achieved her goal of financial independence.

The Indian Territory had passed one of the earliest laws granting full licenses to osteopathic physicians in 1903, and in a region where most of the residents were men working the oil fields, many of the early doctors were women. Dr. Wilkins set up a practice in the oil town of Sapulpa, where she met Bates B. (B. B.) Burnett and his brother, Birch C. Burnett, young bankers who she helped to divert funds from customer accounts to their own. Eventually the brothers were caught and in 1913 they were prosecuted for embezzlement. By then, Dr. Wilkins had learned her lesson—don't trust banks—and moved on.

In about 1910, Dr. Wilkins set up a medical practice in Tulsa, where she married again, this time to a successful furniture dealer who soon left her, taking what few portable assets he had left. Zeo's next lover was a pharmacist from Kansas City whom she had met while practicing in Claremore (30 miles from Tulsa), which was known for its healing springs. She provided him with her own special medical treatments and he gave her fifteen thousand dollars, which was all the money he had. In her diary, she recorded, "He gave me all his money and went to get more…poor man." The "poor man" had shot himself.[83]

Wildcatters struck oil in Claremore in 1912, but it was the healing springs that attracted Thomas W. Cunningham, a wealthy banker from Joplin, Missouri. He was also elderly, widowed, and childless. Cunningham met Zeo when he visited Dr. Wilkins' exclusive medical clinic for a neurological condition that responded well to osteopathic treatment. Once Zeo was sure of her latest conquest, she closed her office in Claremore and moved to Kansas City, where she bought a house with Cunningham's money and advertised her services as an osteopath. Over the next two years, they carried on a long-distance relationship, during which Cunningham gave Zeo about $200,000. Then Zeo decided she should marry the old man. In 1914, they traveled to Gallatin, Missouri, and were quietly married in a private ceremony before returning to Kansas City and taking up residence in the fanciest hotel in town. Cunningham lavished more of his assets on his new bride and she busied herself with transferring his property to her name. In 1916, perhaps concerned about the validity of their marriage, Zeo took Cunningham to Colorado Springs where they went through another marriage ceremony. As a wedding present, the old man gave his bride his stock in the bank. She promptly sold it to a rival bank.[84]

Their marital bliss did not last long. Cunningham's friends from Joplin had become concerned about his extended absence and came looking for him, and back in Joplin, Mrs. Tabitha Taylor, age 72, claimed to be the common-law wife of the old banker and sued for alimony. Zeo found a lawyer to represent her husband in Mrs. Taylor's case against him and another to represent her interests. Meanwhile, Cunningham's friends, convinced that Zeo had bewitched him to the point of insanity, hired lawyers and had the old man taken into protective custody on an insanity warrant. As the lawyers wrangled over what remained of Cunningham's fortune, the newspapers tried to outdo each other with sensational stories of the love triangle of the old millionaire, his aging, common-law wife, and the young siren. Eventually, the cases were settled and Zeo's marriage to Cunningham was annulled; she got to keep most of the property and money he had given her.

In the spring of 1917, Dr. Wilkins returned to her home in Colorado Springs and Albert Marksheffel, a car dealer who was young (only four years older than Zeo) and handsome, but not wealthy. They had started their affair while Zeo was still married to Cunningham. Within months of Zeo's divorce from Cunningham, Albert became husband number five. The marriage to Albert was different however; Zeo gave him money to build the biggest automobile garage in the country and paid for an expensive honeymoon trip. Albert, on the other hand, never gave Zeo the gifts she was accustomed to receiving from husbands and lovers. She asked him to at least bring her flowers but he refused. Once, she took to her bed for three days feigning illness, in an attempt to get his sympathy. When this failed Zeo faked her own death. The ruse was so convincing that Albert fainted from fright. From that time on, he frequently brought her flowers. That is, until Zeo divorced him in 1919.

For the next several years, Dr. Wilkins ran an osteopathic practice in Kansas City, catering to the rich and elite members of society, with an overwhelmingly male clientele. Her practice grew quickly and she was well known in social circles. She continued to accept gifts from wealthy admirers and to invest in oil fields. Her business dealings became shadier than usual and she lost significant amounts of money through bad investments and litigation. On the side she was involved in bootlegging with, among others, her brother Arthur, and may have also been involved with drugs. At least once she was caught in a raid on a speakeasy, and was involved in another lawsuit resulting from an affair with a married man. In 1922, during an extended visit to her sister Gertrude, who ran a sanitarium in Fort Worth, Texas, Zeo had some encounters with the local police and her sister tried to have her treated at her sanitarium. After witnessing several dramatic, but unsuccessful, suicide attempts, Gertrude gave up and Zeo returned to Kansas City.

Dr. Zeo Wilkins opened an osteopathic practice in a rented house in 1922. Earlier that year, she had traveled to Kirksville for an advanced class in "the Abrams method," a new medical treatment that was quickly discredited. Zeo, however, charged high rates for "electric treatments" and continued to build her clientele. When not collecting exorbitant fees for osteopathic treatments, Dr. Wilkins entertained a steady stream of lovers and, for a fee, allowed adulterous couples to use her home as a "trysting place." Despite her apparently successful medical practice, Dr. Wilkins continued to have financial problems.[85]

In fall 1923, Dr. Wilkins was ill and sought treatment from fellow osteopath Dr. Klepinger, who told her she must stop drinking. She called on her brother Charlie to help her and the next months were filled with squabbles and even physical fights among Zeo, Charlie, and her various friends and lovers. On several occasions, she told friends and even the police that she was afraid for her life. On 19 March 1924, Dr. Wilkins was found dead on the floor of her medical office. Her neck had been slashed from ear to ear. The police report indicated that she had put up a great struggle before being killed, and there was a large burnt area in the carpet where her murderer had apparently attempted to burn down her office to cover any clues.[86]

Zeo's diary and other documents showed that Dr. Wilkins had been doing much more than just practicing medicine. Her wealthy male patients would bring

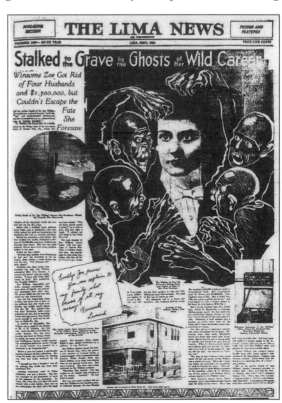

The reporters of her time treated the flamboyant, beautiful osteopath as the paparazzi treat celebrities and royals of today; she loved the attention. [Museum Collection, MOM]

their pregnant mistresses to her; Dr. Wilkins would perform abortions in her office, then blackmail the couple to keep their secret. Many of her male patients had been her lovers and she used this information to solicit funds from them. She had also been peddling drugs. The scandalous life and mysterious murder of Zeo Wilkins made the national and even international news, and reports that diamonds, securities, and hundreds of thousands of dollars were missing from Dr. Wilkins' home and office excited speculation and rumor. Three separate suspects were arrested and even her attorney, Jesse James Jr., son of the famous outlaw, was suspected, but all were eventually released for insufficient evidence and her murder has never been solved.[87]

Isabelle Brake, DO

Isabelle Brake was introduced to osteopathy through her father, James Hugh Brake, an Australian parliamentarian whose sister suffered from a hip condition. Seeking a cure for his sister, the senior Brake took his sister to Europe, along with Isabelle and her brother, James. The Brakes were seeking the services of an Austrian surgeon known for his "bloodless surgery," a term frequently used at the time to describe manipulation, when they heard of the work Dr. Still was doing in Missouri.[88] The particulars of the case are not known, but apparently Dr. Still was so successful that Mr. Brake enrolled both Isabelle and James in the ASO, from which they graduated in 1907.

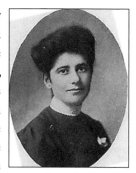

Isabelle Brake, DO
[1907 *Osteoblast*, MOM]

This is another example of the many men and women of the era who devoted their lives to osteopathy after witnessing medicine being practiced without the brutal surgery and toxic medications commonly used at that time.

Isabelle and James returned to Melbourne, where they practiced osteopathy in the Cornhill Building on 450 Collins Street. In the professional and trade section of the 1911 directory of Victoria, five osteopaths were listed as practicing from this site—three of them were women: Isabelle Brake, DO; Florence Mac-George, DO; and Emeline Tappan, DO (ASO, 1901). Edgar Culley, DO (ASO, 1901, and husband of Dr. Tappan) and his brother, Albert B. Culley, DO, made up the group. Isabelle Brake died in 1972.[89]

J. Louise Mason, DO

Louise Mason graduated from the Massachusetts College of Osteopathy in 1911 and from the Los Angeles College of Osteopathy in 1912. While practicing in

Boston in 1918, she answered a call from the American Committee for Relief in the Near East for relief workers in Turkey. She was rejected by the medical unit because she was an osteopath, but her desire to help her fellow man was so strong that she accepted an administrative position. After her return, she wrote two articles about her experiences.

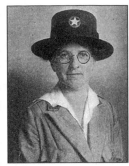

J. Louise Mason, DO, first to bring osteopathy to Asia Minor. [1920 *Osteopathic Physician*, MOM]

On the trip to Turkey, although there was a medical unit in the group, Dr. Mason was frequently called on to administer to the medical needs of the 250 members of the expedition. After a brief stay in Constantinople (modern-day Istanbul), Dr. Mason was assigned to the Trebizond unit with six other relief workers. The unit was to care for the Greek and Armenian widows and children who were returning to the ravaged city after surviving the massacres of Armenians and deportations of Greeks. The Turkish army had destroyed all homes except the ones they were occupying. The only medical care available for the town was Dr. Mason, a nurse with the relief unit, and a local Greek physician who, much to Dr. Mason's liking, prescribed few drugs.[90]

Dr. Mason was in charge of the relief unit and it was her duty to distribute relief supplies and money to the refugees. She established a dispensary, which according to the regulations of the relief organization, was placed under the direction of the nurse. Dr. Mason organized sanitation crews composed of refugee women to clean up the streets of the city; the women were paid for their work.

Dr. Mason also built a homemade osteopathic treatment table from salvaged materials. Although she limited her treatment to children, many of whom had malaria, there were still too many patients to be treated by one person. She used osteopathic manipulation and nutrition, since malnutrition was widespread before the arrival of Dr. Mason and the relief unit. The only medicine available to her was a limited supply of quinine pills. She kept notes and found that 70 percent of malaria patients who came regularly for two weeks or more benefited or were cured. When the American quinine pills ran out, Dr. Mason purchased quinine salts from Constantinople and made her own pills, but noted that the patients preferred the American product.[91]

Dr. Mason wrote that adults would often come in with the children when they were being treated and ask, "What is she doing?" and another would answer, "She is pulling things and putting them in their right places."[92] Dr. Mason worked for ten months in Turkey before being rotated back to America where she resumed her practice of osteopathic medicine in Boston.

Margaret Jones, DO

Margaret Jones graduated from the Kansas City College of Osteopathy and Surgery in 1922. She became the first female osteopathic physician to serve a preceptorship in surgery and was the first woman to be board certified in general surgery by the AOA and the American Osteopathic Board of Surgery.

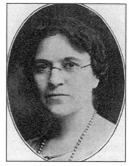

Margaret Jones, DO
[Kansas City University of Medicine and Bioscience]

In 1934, Dr. Jones became the founding president of the American College of Osteopathic Obstetricians and Gynecologists. She served two years as president and then continued to serve on the board of directors for several years. Dr. Jones taught obstetrics and gynecology at the Kansas City College of Osteopathy and Surgery for thirty-three years. She also lectured extensively and authored many articles on obstetrics and gynecology.[93] It would be forty years before another woman, Betty Jo White, DO, would complete an AOA-approved residency in surgery to become the second female osteopathic surgeon.[94]

Olga Gross, DO

Olga Gross graduated from the ASO in 1923 and practiced in Pittsfield, Maine. In addition to her office practice, she was active in athletic medicine as the team physician for the Maine Central Institute, a coeducational preparatory school, serving as the physician for both the male and female athletic teams. Several of the team members she treated went on to become Olympic athletes.

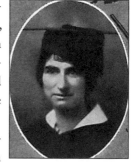

Olga Gross, DO
[1924 *Osteoblast*, MOM]

In the November 1933 issue of *The Osteopathic Profession*, Dr. Gross published an article entitled, "For Men Only? Active Scope for Practice Offered to Women in the Care of School Athletes," in which she encouraged other female osteopathic physicians to participate in athletics as team physicians. She indicated that the young athletes were a source of future patient referrals. Dr. Gross's experience showed that "The school's hospital bills have almost been wiped out since the team has had osteopathic care."[95]

Helen Cottrell Hampton, DO, and the Cottrell/Hampton Osteopathic Dynasty

Andrew Taylor Still's brothers, children, grandchildren, and other family members became osteopaths in the early years of the profession, making them the first osteopathic family dynasty, but they were not the only such dynasty. Throughout the years there have been numerous families dedicated to the profession. One of those dynasties started with Helen Cottrell.

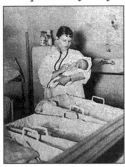

Helen Cottrell was born in Chesterland, Ohio, on 27 June 1900, the daughter of Dr. Mead and Gertrude Cottrell. Helen's father, Mead Kelly Cottrell, DO, graduated from the ASO in 1905 (he was a classmate of Zeo Wilkins). After graduating, he moved to New York

Helen Cottrell Hampton, DO
[Donald Hampton II, DO]

where he practiced for three years before moving to Cleveland, Ohio. When he applied for reciprocity of his New York osteopathic license to Ohio, he was refused. Dr. Cottrell filed suit against the Ohio licensing board and won, thus setting legal precedent for future osteopathic physicians.

Helen grew up around osteopathy. After obtaining a bachelor's degree in dietetics and institutional management, she did the only natural thing and followed in the footsteps of her physician father. After graduating from the ASO in 1923, Helen married Donald Vernon Hampton, a classmate who received his DO degree in 1925 from the Kirksville College of Osteopathy and Surgery.[96] Helen completed an internship at the ASO Hospital so she could be close to her new husband while he was still in school. Drs. Helen and Donald Hampton went into practice with Helen's father in the Commonwealth Building at Euclid Avenue and East 102nd Street in Cleveland, now the location of The Cleveland Clinic's Outpatient Service Building.

Dr. Helen Cottrell Hampton became the first female board-certified osteopathic pediatrician and a founding member of the College of Osteopathic Pediatricians. She went on to become the third president and first female president of this pediatric organization. In the meantime, her husband, Dr. Donald Hampton, was active in the AOA and served as its president in 1952.

Helen and Donald's son, Donald V. Hampton II, graduated from the Kirksville College of Osteopathic Medicine in 1954 and set up his medical practice in Chesterland, Ohio, where his mother had been born. Dr. Donald Hampton II is presently clinical professor emeritus and prior course director of Osteopathic Principles and Practice at the Lake Erie College of Osteopathic Medicine. He teaches at both the Erie, Pennsylvania, and Bradenton, Florida, campuses. His brother, Robert Hampton, graduated from the Ohio University College of Osteopathic Medicine in 1984 and is board certified in orthopedic surgery. He practices in Cleveland, Ohio. Dr. Donald Hampton's niece, Dr. Leslie Buttler, is a board certified osteopathic forensic pathologist, and her husband, Dr. Jeff Buttler is a board-certified osteopathic emergency physician. They practice in Bakersfield, California.[97]

Anna Northup-Little, DO

Anna Northup graduated from the ASO in 1915. She became a pioneer of osteopathy in Canada, establishing her practice in Moose Jaw, Saskatchewan. In the severe Canadian winters, she often made house calls to her patients, frequently plowing through snow drifts to get to them.

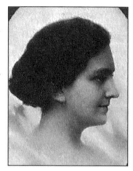

Anna Northup-Little, DO
[1915 *Osteoblast*, MOM]

In 1922, Northup married Alfred Little, a widower with two children, and from then on she was known as Northup-Little. They had a son in 1923 and later adopted a daughter. In 1953, she moved her practice to Regina and joined with Dr. Dorothy Tanner. In recognition of her work for equality for women, the Quota Club of Regina named Dr. Northup-Little Quota Woman of the Year.

Dr. Northup-Little was an organizer and president of the Canadian Osteopathic Association and the Saskatchewan Society of Osteopathic Physicians.[98] She also served as the third vice president of the AOA from 1928 to 1929.[99]

Ruth Elizabeth Tinley, DO

After earning a bachelor's degree in education, Ruth Tinley graduated from the Philadelphia College of Osteopathy in 1923. Dr. Tinley was a well-known pediatrician in Philadelphia, where she practiced her entire professional career until her death in 1963. She was a professor and chairperson of the department of pediatrics and was the director of the children's clinics at the Spring Garden Street and the 48th and Spruce Street hospitals. She was only the second woman ever to chair a department and the first woman to chair the department of pediatrics at the Philadelphia College of Osteopathy.

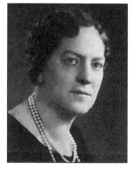

Ruth E. Tinley, DO
[1932 *Synapsis*, PCOM]

Among Dr. Tinley's many accomplishments was serving a term as president of the American Association of Osteopathic Pediatricians. After retiring from the college in 1945, Dr. Tinley remained actively involved with its alumni association.[100]

Ruth Emery, DO

Ruth Emery graduated from the Kirksville College of Osteopathy and Surgery in 1926. After practicing for two years in Saco, Maine, she moved her office to Portland, Maine, where she continued her practice.

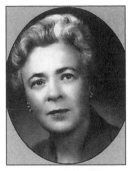

In 1932, Dr. Louise M. Jones joined Dr. Emery's practice. Three years later, Drs. Emery and Jones became part of a group of eleven osteopathic physicians, five women and six men, who founded the Osteopathic Hospital of Maine. During most of their professional lives, Drs. Emery and Jones were members of the board of trustees of the hospital and continued to maintain their very active medical practices. In 1965, the Osteopathic Hospital of Maine honored Dr. Emery for her many years

Ruth Emery, DO
[Osteopathic Hospital of Maine/ Brighton Medical Center]

of dedicated service to the community and the hospital. Dr. Jones died in 1968; Dr. Emery continued to actively practice until her retirement in 1971.[101]

Anne Wales, DO

Anne Wales was born in Cranston, Rhode Island, in 1904. She entered the ASO in 1922 as one of ten women in the class. She transferred to the Kansas City College of Osteopathy and Surgery, where she graduated in 1926. While still in school, she taught the head and neck portion of gross anatomy to the first-year students. When a terrible flu hit the Midwest in the winter of 1925, Anne and her classmates made

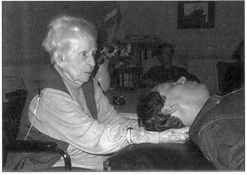

Anne Wales, DO, administering osteopathic manipulative therapy in 2005, shortly after her 101st birthday, while teaching osteopathic cranial techniques to a group of osteopathic physicians.
[Jane Carreiro, DO]

house calls in the local communities. Anne's father had given her the use of his Model T Ford for the winter but had not shown her how to drive it. Using her own resourcefulness, Anne taught herself to drive the Model T and used the car to make house calls while most of the other students used horse and buggy.

From 1926 to 1927 Anne served her internship at Lakeside Hospital in Kansas City. In 1927 she returned to Rhode Island, where she would practice for the next fifty years. Anne Wales was the first woman to take and pass the Rhode Island Osteopathic Licensing Examination. She then spearheaded the campaign to establish the first osteopathic hospital in the state. Although she did this during the Great Depression, patients in the community supported the campaign enthusiastically. In 1933, while still in the midst of the Depression, the Osteopathic Hospital of Rhode Island was opened with Dr. Wales serving as the chief of pediatrics. Although patients were often unable to pay for their care, they were never turned away. As the economy floundered, doctors closed their offices and began practicing out of their homes. In 1938, Dr. Wales closed her office and converted a spare bedroom in her house into a treatment room. A desk in the living room served as the reception area. A colleague, Chester Handy, DO, rented the one-bedroom apartment downstairs and treated patients from there.

In 1942, Dr. Wales and Chester Handy married and used their honeymoon to attend the AOA convention in New York City. There they heard a speech by William Sutherland, DO, the founder of cranial manipulation, that changed Dr. Wales' practice for the rest of her long and productive life.

The first official course of instruction in cranial osteopathy was held at the Des Moines College of Osteopathy and Surgery in 1945. The Academy of Applied Osteopathy formed a committee to assist Dr. Sutherland with his teaching and Dr. Wales was a member. The committee eventually became the Osteopathic Cranial Academy; Dr. Wales assisted in drafting the original bylaws and constitution and served on the board of trustees until 1953. Dr. Wales continued to study and teach the concepts of Dr. Sutherland. She served on his faculty and in 1954 wrote the teacher's guide for the first course taught without Dr. Sutherland.

In 1952, Dr. Wales and her husband established a free osteopathic clinic for handicapped children and their siblings. This free clinic ran successfully in Providence, Rhode Island, until 1964, when Dr. Wales moved to Tiverton, Rhode Island, where she was instrumental in establishing a nursery school for children with mental handicaps. She developed legislative guidelines for the state of Rhode Island to support the care of children with congenital disorders. In time this led to the establishment of the Meeting Street School, the Ladd School, and the Rhode Island School for the Deaf.

In 1961, Dr. Wales edited *Contributions of Thought: The Collected Writings of William Sutherland*. She wrote many articles and papers in the *Journal of the Osteopathic Cranial Association* and the *Journal of the American Osteopathic Association*. She also taught for the Sutherland Cranial Teaching Foundation, lecturing throughout the United States and Europe. In 1981, Dr. Wales retired and moved to Massachusetts; however, her retirement did not last long. To many osteopathic physicians, Dr. Wales was a living legend and she was often asked to share her knowledge with others. She became the director of the Still-Sutherland Study Group, editing *Teachings in the Science of Osteopathy*, and lecturing to fellows, students, residents, and physicians. She frequently said that the later years of her life were some of her happiest. Throughout her lifetime, Dr. Wales received numerous honors and awards and maintained the deep esteem of her fellow physicians.[102]

NOTES

1. Violette, *History of Adair County*, 250–53.

2. "Osteopathy: A. T. Still Infirmary and School Building," [Kirksville] *Democrat*, Sept. 14, 1894.

3. "A Modern Wonder," *Journal of Osteopathy* 2, no. 6 (Sept. 1895): 7.

4. Wabash Railroad advertisement, 1897, MOM.

5. "Located in Kirksville, Missouri," *Journal of Osteopathy* 2, no. 10 (Feb. 1896). 8.

6. Walter, *First School of Osteopathic Medicine*, 54–55.

7. Ibid., 39.

8. Perloff, *To Secure Merit*, 21.

9. "Infirmary and School Notes," *Journal of Osteopathy* 3, no. 2 (July 1896): 4; and "A. T. Still Infirmary," *Journal of Osteopathy* 4, no. 2 (June 1897): frontispiece.

10. Walter, *First School of Osteopathic Medicine*, 14.

11. Gevitz, *The DOs*, 44; Booth, *History of Osteopathy*, 103, 106; Walter, *First School of Osteopathic Medicine*, 32–33; and Trowbridge, *Andrew Taylor Still*, 169–71.

12. Gevitz, *The DOs*, 48.

13. Walter *First School of Osteopathic Medicine*, 45–49.

14. Ibid., 45–49; and Gevitz, *The DOs*, 52.

15. "Ward Sole Owner of CSO," [Kirksville] *Democrat*, 19 Jan. 1900; and Walter, *First School of Osteopathic Medicine*, 47.

16. Gevitz, *The DOs*, 48.

17. The World Osteopathic Health Organization (www.woho.org) defines an osteopathic physician as "A person with full, unlimited medical practice rights who has achieved the nationally recognized academic and professional standards within her or his country to independently practice, diagnose, and provide treatment based upon the principles of osteopathic philosophy." The World Osteopathic Health Organization defines an osteopath as "A person who has achieved the nationally recognized academic and professional standards within her or his country to independently practice, diagnose, and provide treatment based

upon the principles of osteopathic philosophy."

18. "Proceedings of the Fifth Annual Meeting of the AAAO," *JAOA* 1 (1901): 6–15; and Hulett, "Historical Sketch of the AAAO," *JAOA* 1 (1900): 1–6.

19. Booth, *History of Osteopathy,* 273.

20. "Constitution of the American Osteopathic Association," *JAOA* 1 (1901): 16–17; "Proceedings of the Fifth Annual Meeting of the AAAO," *JAOA* 1 (1901): 6–15; and Booth, *History of Osteopathy,* 115, 251.

21. Kett, *Formation of the American Medical Profession,* 23.

22. Gevitz, *The DOs,* 55, 65.

23. "ASO to Adopt Three Year Course," *Journal of Osteopathy* 12, no. 1 (Jan. 1905): 1.

24. Gevitz, *The DOs,* 28–29, 45.

25. American Osteopathic Association, *Yearbook and Directory, 1913,* 169–89; and American Osteopathic Association, *Yearbook and Directory, 1923,* 97–108.

26. Booth, *History of Osteopathy,* 81.

27. *Toledo Times,* 14 May 1902, quoted in Booth, *History of Osteopathy,* 168.

28. "Some Foolish Things to Be Dropped," *Journal of Osteopathy* 10, no. 4 (April 1903): 8.

29. Patterson, "Why Not Call Our Women Doctors?" *Journal of Osteopathy* 12, no. 12 (Dec. 1907): 18.

30. Crosby, *Epidemic and Peace,* 206–7.

31. Booth, *History of Osteopathy,* 115.

32. Gevitz, *The DOs,* 84.

33. "Proceedings of the House of Delegates," *Forum of Osteopathy* 3 (Aug. 1929): supp. 5–8.

34. *Flexner Report,* 137, 158.

35. Gevitz, *The DOs,* 83–90.

36. Jones, *The Difference a D.O. Makes,* 23. For an osteopathic appreciation of Flexner's reform advocacy, see "Imaginative Vision and Organizational Capacity," *JAOA* 56 (May 1957): 549–50.

37. *Flexner Report,* 163.

38. Gevitz, *The DOs,* 89.

39. Walter, *First School of Osteopathic Medicine,* 59–64.

40. Armstrong and Armstrong, *Great American Medicine Show,* 3, 10–11, 35–37, 144.

41. Perloff, *To Secure Merit,* 11.

42. Klofkorn and Dodson, *One Hundred Years of Osteopathic Medicine,* 56.

43. "From President Willard: Materia Medica," *JAOA* 25 (Dec. 1925): 279–80.

44. American Osteopathic Association, "Historic Reference of Osteopathic Colleges," accessed 18 Feb. 2011, http://history.osteopathic.org/collegehist.shtml.

45. *Flexner Report,* 178.

46. Ibid., 179.

47. Simpson and Weiser, "Studying the Impact of Women on Osteopathic Physician Workforce Predictions," *JAOA* 96, no. 2 (Feb. 1996): 107–8.

48. Walter, *Women and Osteopathic Medicine,* 20–21.

49. Smith, "What the OWNA Is Doing for Osteopathy," *Clinical Osteopathy* (April 1940): 226–29.

50. McNeff, "The Women's Challenge," *Forum of Osteopathy* 2, no. 8 (Nov. 1928): 8.

51. Untitled manuscript [1999.10, 2010.02] Alice Patterson-Shibley, DO, Collection, MOM.

52. Hildreth, *Lengthening Shadow of Dr. Andrew Taylor Still,* 41.

53. Walter, *First School of Osteopathic Medicine,* 30–31.

54. Walter, *Women and Osteopathic Medicine,* 11–12.

55. "Female Leaders of the AOA," 28.

56. Gevitz, *The DOs,* 51–52.

57. Booth, *History of Osteopathy,* 167.

58. Gevitz, *The DOs,* 51–52.

59. Booth, *History of Osteopathy,* 86–87, 166–67.

60. Walter, *Women and Osteopathic Medicine,* 15; and Fitzgerald, "Women in History, Pioneers of the Profession," *The DO* 25 (Dec. 1984): 67–71.

61. Hulett, "Historical Sketch of the AAAO," *JAOA* 1 (1900): 1–6; and "Female Leaders of the AOA," 25.

62. Walter, *First School of Osteopathic Medicine,* 186–87; "Des Moines Funds New College," *Osteopathic Physician* 8, no. 3 (June 1905): 1; and Hildreth, *Lengthening Shadow of Andrew Taylor Still,* 203.

63. Walter, *First School of Osteopathic Medicine,* 81, 99–101.

64. Letter, Minnie F. Potter to T. L. Ray, unnumbered, MOM.

65. Grace, *Carry A. Nation,* 131; and Nation, *Use and Need of the Life of Carrie A. Nation,* 70, 133.

66. Letter to the editor, *Barbar County Index,* 1900.

67. Personal library of A. T. Still, MOM.

68. Perloff, *To Secure Merit,* 4.

69. Letter of Mrs. Marion W. Jenks, 169, quoted in ibid.

70. *The Nucleolus,* 1911, pp. 115–16; "Deaths," *Forum of Osteopathy* 27 (Nov. 1952): 261; and "Locations and Removals," *Journal of Osteopathy* 17 (Dec. 1910): 1250.

71. "Female Leaders of the AOA," 28; "Editorials," *Journal of Osteopathy* 21 (May 1914): 302; and "Change of Editors," *Journal of Osteopathy* 21 (Aug. 1914): 499.

72. "Book Reviews," *Journal of Osteopathy* 23 (Jan. 1916): 58; and "A Practical Text-Book on 'Osteopathic Mechanics' Has at Last Been Produced!!!" *Osteopathic Physician* 30, no. 2 (Feb. 1916): 1.

73. Conger, *Ohio Woman in the Philippines,* 23.

74. Fox, "Emily Bronson Conger, 1843–1917," *Akron Women's History,* accessed 8 Nov., 2006, http://www.uakron.edu/schlcomm/womenshistory/conger_e.htm.

75. Florence MacGeorge, DO, Handwritten manuscript, undated, untitled, D792, MOM.

76. Who's Who, "Unusual Honor for Dr. Morelock," *Forum of Osteopathy* 1, no. 5 (Aug. 1927): 22.

77. Bunting, "Science Offers New Field for the Blind," *Journal of Osteopathy* 5, no. 10 (March 1899): 490.

78. Carson, Open letter, *Journal of Osteopathy* 26, no. 12 (Dec. 1919): 760.

79. Veazie, Open letter, *Journal of Osteopathy* 26, no. 12 (Dec. 1919): 760.

80. Dr. Wilkins's story appeared in Anton Booker's 1945 *Wildcats in Petticoats,* and in Bernard O'Donnell's 1990 "The Vampire of Kansas City" in Sebastian Wolfe, ed., *Kiss and Kill.* Most recently, Laura James published *The Love Pirate and the Bandit's Son,* a carefully researched book on Zeo Wilkins and Jesse James Jr. While contemporary newspaper

stories and previous accounts contain contradictions on many details, James has evaluated the conflicting sources and written a reliable account of the life of Zeo Wilkins. This brief summary is drawn primarily from James's work. Additional sources found in Wilkins' biographical file at MOM are listed in the notes.

81. Quote from "Zeo Z. Wilkins is Slain," *Kansas City Times*[?], 19 March 1924, in Wilkins biographical file, MOM. This article gives his name as "Richard Dryder."

82. "Stalked to the Grave by the Ghosts of Her Wild Career," *Lima* (Ohio) *News*, in Wilkins biographical file, MOM.

83. O'Donnell, "Vampire of Kansas City," 219.

84. "In a Tangle," *Chicago Tribune*, February 1917; and "Zeo's Diary Bares Life," newspaper clipping, both in Wilkins biographical file, MOM.

85. "Zoe Wilkins' Will Sought; Brother Held," *Chicago Daily Tribune*, 20 March 1924, in Wilkins biographical file, MOM.

86. Ibid.

87. Ibid.

88. Hawkins and O'Neill, *Osteopathy in Australia*, 19–20.

89. Ibid.

90. Mason, "Osteopathy Cures Patients in Turkey," *JAOA* 19 (March 1920): 242.

91. Mason, "An Osteopath in Turkey," *Journal of Osteopathy* 28, no. 4 (April 1921): 232–35.

92. Ibid., 235.

93. Information on Dr. Margaret Jones from Richard Polk, DO, Clinical Professor Emeritus OSU-COM, personal correspondence to author, 4 December 2006.

94. Burnett, "Women Contribute Greatly to Medicine: Andrew Taylor Still Memorial Address," *The DO* (Oct. 1999): 56.

95. Gross, "For Men Only? Active Scope for Practice Offered to Women in the Care of School Athletes," *Osteopathic Profession* 1 (Nov. 1933): 33.

96. The American School of Osteopathy changed its name to the Kirksville College of Osteopathy and Surgery in 1924.

97. Information on Dr. Helen Cottrell Hampton and her family from Donald Hampton II, DO, personal correspondence with the author, 6 October 2006.

98. Information on Anna Northup supplied by Ted Findley, president of the Canadian Osteopathic Association, personal correspondence with the author, 18 December 2006.

99. *JAOA* (Sept. 1928): 18.

100. Perloff, *To Secure Merit*, 35.

101. Parker, *Historical Memoirs*, 16, 21–23.

102. Information on Dr. Anne Wales from Jane Carreiro, DO, personal correspondence with author, 21 December 2007.

Chapter Four

*T*he Middle Years of Osteopathic Medicine, 1930–1964

"In placing women among physicians, Dr. Still has put them back in the place they occupied a few centuries ago when the great lady with her herbs and simples was the physician of the feudal times."

Jeanette "Nettie" Bolles, DO

"When a cat gets his tail in a door, don't say 'poor kitty', or try to appease its pain by petting it. Open the door and let it loose. You are Osteopaths and thus get at the cause."

Andrew Taylor Still, MD, DO

DURING THE EARLY YEARS OF THE PROFESSION when the American Osteopathic Association (AOA) and the Associated Colleges of Osteopathy were established as the accrediting agencies for the osteopathic profession, they accredited only those osteopathic colleges that taught a standardized curriculum.[1] But what about those DOs trained in the diploma mills who were still in practice? They still existed, held limited licenses, and could call themselves DOs. By 1925, all graduating osteopathic physicians in the United States were products of schools approved by the AOA and the Associated Colleges of Osteopathy,[2] and by 1931, four years after their joint mandate passed in 1927, all osteopathic graduates were fully trained on an equal basis with the allopathic schools, including *materia medica* (pharmaceuticals).[3]

As the years passed, more fully trained DOs graduated and more of the partially licensed and diploma-mill doctors retired. The profession worked hard, state by state, to obtain full, unrestricted licensure for the fully trained DOs. The American Medical Association (AMA), however, continued to classify all osteopaths, including the fully trained and licensed osteopathic physicians, as "cultists" and to declare that it was "unethical" for any licensed MD to work with or consult with a DO.[4]

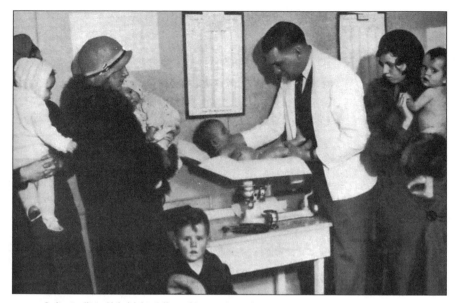

Pediatrics Clinic, Philadelphia College of Osteopathy, with Leo C. Wagner, DO, 1933. The clinic provided much-needed medical care to medically underserved areas during the great depression. [PCOM 1996.549]

The AOA and the osteopathic profession also worked diligently to update the public perception of osteopathic medicine as a complete form of medical practice and to update the definitions of osteopathic medicine in dictionaries and encyclopedias.[5]

Although most of the reforms in medical education made by MD-granting schools occurred during the first twenty-five years after the release of the Flexner Report, the smaller osteopathic medical schools, with their more limited financing and resources, made the most of their reforms during the second twenty-five years after the release of the report.[6] The AOA mandated that all accredited osteopathic medical schools have a minimum entrance requirement of one year of college education by 1938 and two years by 1940.[7] By 1954, the minimum entrance requirement for all osteopathic colleges was three years of college, and by 1960, over 70 percent of entering osteopathic medical students had a bachelor's degree, with many having advanced degrees.[8]

Because osteopathic physicians were routinely denied permission to work in allopathic hospitals, the osteopathic profession was forced to develop its own hospital system;[9] however, because of the sparse distribution of osteopathic physicians, with many DOs providing care to rural and medically underserved areas, it was difficult to find clusters of DOs in sufficient numbers to open anything but small osteopathic hospitals. And because DOs understandably tended to avoid areas where it was difficult or impossible to obtain full medical licensure, there were areas of the country where osteopathy was virtually unknown.[10] Many of the early osteopathic hospitals were opened in converted homes or mansions and, unlike allopathic hospitals, none received government subsidies. They relied solely on the money the hospitals could generate and on donations from within the profession. Although small by allopathic standards, most of these osteopathic facilities were full-service hospitals providing medical, surgical, obstetrical, pediatric, and emergency services.

In the 1940s, many large health insurance companies, with MDs dominating their governing boards and under pressure from the AMA, refused to cover care for their policyholders who chose osteopathic hospitals,[11] and this was before the era of "managed care" when insurance companies began offering lower-cost policies by restricting care to a particular network of physicians and/or hospitals. Because insurance companies were incorporated under state charters, the osteopathic profession was forced to undertake a state-by-state campaign to compel the payment of legitimate medical bills of policyholders who received care from osteopathic physicians.[12]

During World War II, many MDs were pressed into military service but osteopathic physicians were refused medical commissions. Despite the 1917 law providing for the commissioning of DOs as medical officers (HR 5407), and further bills passed in 1941 (PL 139) and 1942 (PL 763), the military hierarchy, under pressure from MDs and the AMA, refused to commission osteopathic physicians.[13] This setback to the profession, however, had a silver lining. The selective service determined that osteopathic physicians were indispensable to maintaining the health of the civilian population and thus were exempt from the draft.[14] The osteopathic hospital system swelled and offices of osteopathic physicians overflowed with patients who previously had no knowledge of osteopathic medicine. When MDs returned from the battlefields, they found that many of their patients had learned the benefits of osteopathic medicine and decided to remain with their DOs. Although the flow of patients into the osteopathic profession was forced upon the American public by the reduced availability of MDs during the war, the choice to remain with DOs was based on patients' positive experiences with osteopathic medicine.[15]

During the war, women throughout the country filled jobs left vacant by men who were serving in the military. Female physicians, both MDs and DOs, filled voids left by their male colleagues. At the same time, women also filled vacant positions in schools, including medical schools.[16] Despite this, osteopathic medical schools, unlike osteopathic hospitals, which grew and flourished during the war, suffered severely. In 1937, there were 1,977 students in eight osteopathic colleges. By 1940, there were only 1,653 students in seven colleges.[17] The Central College of Osteopathy in Kansas City, Missouri, had closed for financial reasons and merged with the Kansas City College of Osteopathy and Surgery. Four years later, as a direct result of the continued loss of students and faculty due to the war effort, the Massachusetts College of Osteopathy also closed, reducing the total osteopathic enrollment to a mere 556 students in six colleges.[18] During the war, the osteopathic profession lost 72 percent of its students and 25 percent of its educational facilities. Finally by 1947, student enrollment at osteopathic colleges had returned to prewar levels and would remain stable for over a decade.[19] Most importantly, for the first time the number of applicants increased to where there were many more applicants than there were seats available, thus making admissions to osteopathic colleges more competitive than ever before.[20] These postwar applicants, however, were overwhelmingly male.

Overall, the medical profession expanded during the postwar period, fueled in part by the baby boom. Expansion of private health insurance and passage of the Hospital Survey and Construction Act of 1946 (Hill-Burton Act)[21] also contributed to the growth. This act provided money to modernize the nation's hospitals, many of which had become obsolete during the Great Depression and World War II.[22] For the first time, osteopathic hospitals were eligible to receive a share of this financing, allowing internship and residency programs in osteopathic hospitals to be expanded until they were sufficient to train all of the graduating osteopathic physicians.

One factor that contributed to the increase in enrollment in osteopathic medical schools was the GI Bill, which provided tuition for eligible veterans. While this led to a general increase in college enrollment, it also led to a proportionate decrease in the enrollment of women in most professional schools during the late 1940s, 1950s, and early 1960s. In *To Secure Merit*, Perloff attributes the decline in female enrollment at the Philadelphia College of Osteopathy to the shifting of the social mores during the postwar period when men who had postponed their education flooded colleges and professional schools, leaving few seats open for women applicants.[23] Shifting social mores also led to gender discrimination. One of the most blatant examples was a 1946 advertisement run by a large New York City hospital in the *Herald Tribune* that stated "Doctors Wanted: Women Need Not Apply." The AOA responded with an article in the *Forum of Osteopathy* entitled "Doctors Wanted: Women Urged to Apply."[24]

This advertisement and article were just a continuation of the long battle between the AMA and osteopathic medicine that stretched back to the turn of the century. For half a century, the AMA had systematically fought against legal recognition of osteopathic medicine and had labeled the profession "a quackish system," referring to osteopathic physicians as "degenerates who constitute most of the devotees of quackery." During those years, MDs fought to deny DOs full medical licensing in many states, then pushed for legal action against individual DOs for practicing medicine without a license. In 1893, Charles Still, son of A. T. Still, was sued by an MD for practicing medicine without a license when he treated diphtheria-stricken children in Red Wing, Minnesota. As part of his defense, Dr. Charles Still showed that of the seventy children he had treated, only one had died, a remarkable success against this deadly disease. When the local population rallied to support Dr. Charles Still, the MD withdrew his lawsuit, realizing the futility of a legal attack on sound medical treatment.[25]

The AMA also distributed incorrect and misleading information to the public in an attempt to discredit the osteopathic profession, intimidated hospitals to prevent them from accepting DOs on their medical staffs, and worked with insurance companies to deny payments for osteopathic medical care. In addition, the AMA in 1923 labeled osteopathic medicine a "cult" and declared it unethical for MDs to consult with DOs. These attacks continued for decades, during which time the AMA made no attempt to examine the principles and practices of the osteopathic profession, while arguing that only physicians holding an MD degree were scientifically qualified medical practitioners.[26]

The AOA fought back, arguing for full medical licensing of osteopathic physicians, insurance coverage for patients of osteopathic physicians, commissioning of DOs as medical officers in the military, and acceptance of DOs on hospital staffs. Finally, a disgruntled group of DOs in California formed the Metropolitan University College of Medicine and Surgery, whose sole purpose was to grant MD degrees to any osteopathic physician who would pay their tuition and attend thirty-six hours of instruction. In 1947 and 1948, this diploma mill issued 137 MD degrees. This scheme was so obviously a fraud that the AOA and the real California MDs, in a rare instance of professional agreement, quickly moved to close down the institution.[27]

In 1952, the AMA finally decided to inspect the osteopathic profession to determine just how scientific or unscientific the profession really was. After numerous meetings between the AMA and the AOA, the inspection was finally approved in December 1954. Five of the six osteopathic medical schools agreed to the AMA inspection of their facilities and educational processes. The Philadelphia College of Osteopathy, concerned that the inspection appeared to be an accreditation process by the AMA, refused to allow the inspection. The following July, the AMA inspection committee presented its report to the AMA House of Delegates, concluding that admissions requirements for osteopathic schools equaled admission requirements of AMA-approved schools; hours of instruction at osteopathic colleges exceeded hours of instruction at AMA-approved schools by several hundred hours; and that osteopathic colleges taught "the acceptance and recognition of all etiological factors and pathological manifestations of disease" and "the same diagnostic and therapeutic procedures taught in schools of medicine."[28] The investigating committee recommended that the AMA declare that osteopathic medicine was not "cultist healing" and remove the prohibition against MDs consulting with DOs or teaching in DO colleges. The AMA House of Delegates, however, ultimately rejected the committee's conclusions,[29] and the AMA continued its persecution of the minority medical profession. In the eyes of the AOA, the AMA's rejection of its own inspection report reinforced the view that the accusation of "cultist" was merely a political tool to suppress the osteopathic profession. The continual harassment sapped the financial reserves of the already underfunded osteopathic profession, and limited its ability to fund osteopathic research and expand the educational system. The growth of osteopathy stagnated, but the profession became resilient as it shored up its defenses.

While the AOA was preoccupied with these struggles with the AMA and the battle to gain recognition as a separate but equal medical profession, female enrollment continued to drop. By the mid-1950s, individuals were calling for the need to recruit female candidates to osteopathy. A 1953 letter in the *Forum of Osteopathy* maintained that "there are too few women coming into our colleges to take the places of those who retire or whom we lose by death."[30] It would be another decade before this trend would start to reverse.

In the meantime, the AMA abruptly changed its tactics. In 1959, the California Medical Association and the California Osteopathic Association (COA) were involved in secret negotiations to merge the two organizations. For decades, a group of California DOs who had trained at the College of Osteopathic Physicians and Surgeons in Los Angeles had believed they were superior to DOs from the rest of the country, in part because they had Los Angeles General Hospital, Unit #2, owned and funded by the state government, providing high quality residency training programs for its students. The institution, which opened in 1928, was adjacent to Unit #1 of the Los Angeles County General Hospital, which was ten times larger and exclusively allopathic. Patients admitted to the hospital were randomly assigned to a unit, with both units receiving a similar range of critically ill patients.[31] Initially, out of every ten patients, nine went to the allopathic Unit #1 and one went to the osteopathic Unit #2, and a common hospital administration gathered and published annual statistics for each unit. The results of the data showed that medical death rates, postsurgical death rates, and infant mortality rates were significantly lower in the osteopathic Unit #2 compared to the allopathic Unit #1, and that the average length of hospitalization in all categories was shorter in the osteopathic unit.[32] Every patient in Unit #2 received osteopathic manipulative treatments and a clinic was available to continue treatments after discharge.[33] By 1931, the osteopathic unit was handling one out of every seven patients because of the shortened length of hospitalization required.[34] From the beginning, the statistics were so embarrassing for the allopathic Unit #1 that in 1934, the MDs insisted that the administration combine the statistics for both units and publish only the combined figures.[35] In 1956, the osteopathic Unit #2 moved into larger facilities, more than tripling the number of beds available,[36] and began providing even more osteopathic residency positions.

In spite of their excellent performance, the California DOs were continually frustrated that they did not receive the same recognition as the MDs. The allopathic medical schools received government funding, but the College of Osteopathic Physicians and Surgeons and other osteopathic medical schools were forced to rely almost exclusively on tuition for funding.[37] The California DOs felt that their education was superior to osteopathic training in other states and that the AOA should force other colleges to raise their standards.[38] The DOs' discontent with the lack of recognition and their real or perceived sense of lower social standing in California created a deep sense of envy directed at California MDs, who looked down on the DOs and wanted nothing more than to rid their state of what they perceived to be lesser physicians.[39]

In June 1959, the AMA, headed by the California delegation, passed a resolution stating, "It shall not be considered contrary to the principals of medical ethics for doctors of medicine to teach students in an osteopathic college which is in the process of being converted into an approved medical school which is under the supervision of the AMA Council on Medical Education and Hospitals."[40] The Judicial Council of the AMA dropped the "cultist" label and made it possible for allopathic physicians to voluntarily associate with osteopathic physicians.[41] This seemingly well-intentioned act was the first visible display of the AMA's new strategy to destroy through assimilation the only remaining type of medicine not controlled by them. In October 1959, at their annual convention, the AOA responded:

"Be it resolved that the osteopathic school of medicine, in the interest of providing the best possible health care to the public, shall maintain its status as a separate and complete school of medicine."[42] The California delegation resolutely opposed the resolution; the osteopathic profession, although accustomed to assaults from outside, was totally unprepared for rebellion within its own ranks.

At that time, there were six osteopathic medical schools in the United States. California had 10 percent of all the practicing DOs in the country and 60 percent of all the osteopathic residency programs in the profession. It had the largest and best financed osteopathic medical school and fifty-nine osteopathic hospitals, the largest number of osteopathic hospitals in any single state.[43] Pennsylvania had the second largest osteopathic college, the only osteopathic medical school on the east coast. The four smaller colleges were clustered in three adjoining states in the Midwest.

The AMA was determined that there should be only one medical profession and that it should be the organization to control all of medicine. In June 1961, the AMA Judicial Council declared, "There cannot be two distinct sciences of medicine or two different yet equally valid systems of medical practice."[44] If the AMA could absorb osteopathic physicians in California and Pennsylvania, it would control the two largest osteopathic colleges and the only osteopathic medical schools on the East and West Coasts, thereby confining osteopathy to Missouri, Illinois, and Iowa.

In 1960, the AOA learned of the clandestine meetings between the California Medical Association and the COA and threatened to revoke the COA's charter. When the COA openly continued merger negotiations, the AOA revoked its charter and organized the Osteopathic Physicians and Surgeons of California, which was composed of loyal DOs.[45] In 1961, the COA announced its merger with the AMA, and the College of Osteopathic Physicians and Surgeons in Los Angeles became an allopathic medical school under the name of the California College of Medicine. The only change in curriculum was to shorten the length of studies by eliminating the osteopathic courses. With the AMA's blessing, the newly reorganized medical school awarded over two thousand MD degrees to California DOs. For only sixty-five dollars, any graduate from the former osteopathic college in Los Angeles or from any other osteopathic college who held a license in the State of California could purchase an MD degree, with the only condition being that they could no longer identify themselves as osteopathic physicians.[46]

This event, which many refer to as the "California merger," can be considered the "osteopathic civil war," with the COA as the rebels who broke with the larger osteopathic community in calling for a merger with allopathic physicians.

The leader of the rebellion was Dorothy Marsh, DO, who was president of the COA in the 1960s. Dr. Marsh was a charismatic physician specializing in obstetrics and gynecology. She was also a well-known motivational speaker who traveled throughout California giving impassioned speeches in an effort to convince DOs to support the merger with MDs. It is difficult to understand what her motives were in betraying her roots and working to destroy the profession that had given her the opportunity to become a physician; however, her dynamic rhetoric convinced the majority of California DOs to surrender their osteopathic identity and join the majority medical community. Just as the allopathic medical community had destroyed and/or assimilated the homeopathic, physiomedical, and eclectic medical communities, Dr. Marsh's signature on the amalgamation document was supposed to mark the end of the osteopathic medical profession.

Emboldened by their success in California, the AMA in June 1961 adopted a new policy allowing each state medical association to determine what relationship would exist between the two medical professions within their own state, essentially adopting a policy of "divide and conquer."[47] The DOs, led by the AOA, started to fight back. The *Journal of the AOA* referred to this purchased degree as the "md" degree, stating that "the [lowercase] type was chosen in accord with the academic stature of the new type of md degree."[48] The AOA was determined to remain independent, but the AMA was just as determined to eliminate its only remaining competition. In 1962, the California Medical Association was successful in having a new law passed to prohibit new DOs from receiving licenses to practice osteopathic medicine in California. There was, however, a group of 260 California osteopathic physicians who refused to accept the paper "md" and would be allowed to continue to practice under the independent osteopathic licensing board until their numbers dropped below forty. At that time, the board would automatically be dissolved and the MD board would control all medical practice in the state.[49] The first phase of the attack was extremely successful for the allopathic physicians and disastrous for the osteopaths. California had fallen to the rebel osteopathic faction and their AMA ally.

In 1962, the AMA was in open negotiations with promerger groups of DOs throughout the country, including Pennsylvania, home of the largest remaining osteopathic college, the Philadelphia College of Osteopathy. If the Pennsylvania merger had been successful, the osteopathic educational system would have been reduced to the four small colleges clustered in a few hundred square miles in the center of the country. The AMA then had only to tighten the noose in order to strangle the profession. In May 1963, the Pennsylvania Osteopathic Association rejected the merger with the Pennsylvania Medical Society, but stated that they would continue "to meet with the [medical society] to discuss any matters of mutual interest, except amalgamation."[50] This was not the end of the osteopathic civil war, but it was the battle that changed the tide of war.

In 1962, a group of discontented osteopaths in the state of Washington broke off from the state osteopathic organization. Forming their own society, they opened negotiations on a merger with the Washington branch of the AMA. The dissenting DOs opened their own MD school, but it was little more than a paper school reminiscent of the diploma mills of the late nineteenth and early twentieth centuries. The school proved to be short lived when the Washington State Supreme Court declared it and the MD degrees it issued to be illegitimate and void.[51]

The California merger that was supposed to be the beginning of the end of the osteopathic profession did not work out as the AMA had planned. In order to achieve the merger in California, the AMA had to remove its label of "cultist" from osteopathic physicians, and in order to grant AMA-approved MD degrees to over two thousand DOs without any additional educational requirements, had to admit that osteopathic training was at least equal to MD training. In order to approve osteopathic hospitals and accept DOs on the staff of exclusively MD hospitals, the AMA had to admit that osteopathic care was at least equal to allopathic care.[52] All of this meant that the AMA could no longer try to prevent full medical licensure for DOs by claiming that osteopathic medical education was incomplete or of a lesser quality. It was particularly embarrassing for MDs to admit that in order for an osteopathic college to become an allopathic college, the only requirement was to reduce the length of study.

The AOA lost no time in utilizing the unexpected effects of the merger to push for full and unlimited medical licensure in the remaining states where the AMA still blocked its efforts. Osteopathic physicians, with the strong backing of the AOA, then worked to end barring DOs from practicing in previously MD-only hospitals. Under pressure, in 1960 the Joint Commission on the Accreditation of Hospitals made it possible for mixed-staff (DO and MD) hospitals and medical institutions to receive accreditation.[53] These actions enabled the osteopathic profession, under the leadership of the AOA, to make marked advances in the public acceptance of the profession.

In California, the new "md" physicians faced several challenges to full acceptance. California MDs welcomed the former osteopathic physicians, who were mostly family physicians, into their hospitals to provide referrals to MD specialists, but the MD profession already had more specialists than it needed and they did not welcome ex-osteopathic specialists, who themselves soon experienced a dramatic loss of referrals because many of the new "md" family doctors started to refer patients to MD specialists. Another problem arose because the existing AMA rules stipulated that to be recognized as a specialist, a physician must have completed a residency at an AMA-approved hospital. This issue had not been addressed in the merger agreement and after the merger there was little motivation on the part of the AMA or California Medical Association to fix the problem. Still another complication arose over problems absorbing all of the ex-DOs into the state's regular forty regional societies. Five years after the merger there were still a significant number of ex-DOs who had not been absorbed into their regional society.[54]

The fifty-nine former osteopathic hospitals in California also fared very poorly, losing many of their referrals as physicians began to refer patients to larger and/or closer allopathic hospitals. At the same time, internship and residency programs in the smaller ex-osteopathic hospitals closed or were transferred to the larger allopathic hospitals. In 1972, a survey of osteopathic physicians was conducted. Fewer than 8 percent of DOs responding felt that "the merger in California was a successful one." Over 92 percent had deemed it to be unsuccessful.[55]

During these middle years, the osteopathic profession had greatly improved the quality of training for its physicians, and by the end of the era, most states were granting unrestricted licenses to DOs. Despite these advances, the number of graduating DOs had greatly decreased. The profession had lost over one-third of the osteopathic medical schools during this period, going from eight schools in 1938 down to five schools in 1962. By 1964 the osteopathic profession was faced with six major problems:

First: The decrease in the number of women entering colleges and professional schools following World War II continued through the 1950s and into the early 1960s. By 1964, the percentage of osteopathic medical students who were women was at its lowest point in the history of the profession.[56]

Second: The number of osteopathic students graduating from the remaining five osteopathic medical schools was so low that the already small profession was dwindling still further.

Third: DOs were still prevented from joining the armed services with full rank and privilege equal to that of MDs.

Fourth: There were still a handful of states that did not grant full, unrestricted practice rights to DOs.

Fifth: The osteopathic hospital system that had surged during World War II was having difficulty maintaining sufficient numbers of staff physicians as the number of graduating osteopathic physicians decreased and some DOs chose to join the medical staffs of previously MD-only hospitals.

Sixth: With the loss of California, the profession had lost over 60 percent of its residency programs, creating a deficit in specialty residency positions for DOs. While the osteopathic profession has always prided itself on training primary care physicians, specialty physicians were needed to staff the osteopathic hospitals. Without these specialty physicians, osteopathic hospitals would soon become limited in their scope of practice.

WOMEN GRADUATING BETWEEN 1930 AND 1964
Ruth Waddel Cathie, DO, MD

Ruth Emanuel graduated from the Philadelphia College of Osteopathy in 1938. After marrying classmate Herman Waddel, she earned her MD degree from Kansas City University, attending classes on a part-time basis. She gained practical experience working with a pathologist for the City of New York and received special training under George Papanicolaou, MD, PhD, inventor of the Pap smear. For several years, she and her husband practiced at the Osteopathic General Hospital in Dumont, New Jersey.

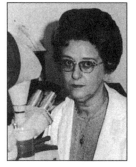

Ruth Waddel Cathie, DO, MD
[1969 *Synapsis*, PCOM]

In 1954, Ruth Waddel joined the faculty at the Philadelphia College of Osteopathy and for the next twenty-one years devoted her life to teaching and practicing pathology at the college and hospital. For seven years she served as professor and chairperson of the Department of Pathology and as director of laboratories at Philadelphia College of Osteopathic Medicine and its hospitals. She was the first woman to chair a basic science department at the college.

Dr. Waddel was widowed in 1963 and in 1969 she married Angus Cathie, DO, the renowned anatomist who had, at the Philadelphia College of Osteopathic Medicine, created one of the most unique anatomy exhibits in the world.

Dr. Waddel Cathie has been honored by the Philadelphia college and the osteopathic profession on many occasions. She received the Christian R. and Mary F. Lindback Foundation Award for Distinguished Teaching as well as the Alumni Association's Certificate of Honor. In 1980, the American Osteopathic College of Pathologists named her Pathologist of the Year. Dr. Waddel Cathie is a past president of the organization and was the first DO allowed to attend the annual lectures of the Armed Forces Institute of Pathology.[57]

Marjorie O. Gutensohn, DO

Marjorie Olwen Gutensohn was born in Melbourne, Australia, and immigrated to the United States. She graduated from the Kirksville College of Osteopathy and Surgery in 1943. She started her practice in North Dakota, but at the end of World War II she and her husband, Max T. Gutensohn, DO, practiced in Melbourne for a year.

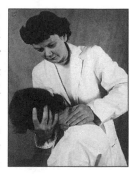

After returning to the United States, Dr. Gutensohn joined the faculty at the Kirksville College of Osteopathy and Surgery as a researcher in physiology and an instructor in neuroanatomy. She also taught osteopathic manipulative therapy. She was board certified in rehabilitation medicine and became a fellow of the College of Rehabilitation Medicine.

Marjorie Olwen Gutensohn, DO
[MOM PH 728]

From 1949 until 1967, Dr. Gutensohn participated in research with Stedman Denslow, DO, a renowned osteopathic researcher. Upon her retirement in 1979, she was named emeritus associate professor of anatomy. Her husband was an emeritus professor of internal medicine. In 1984, the Kirksville College of Osteopathic Medicine dedicated the Gutensohn Osteopathic Health and Wellness Clinic in honor of Drs. Max and Olwen Gutensohn for their long service and dedication to the college and to osteopathic medicine.[58]

Louise Astell, DO

Louise Astell graduated from the Kirksville College of Osteopathy and Surgery in 1945. She established a practice of osteopathic medicine in Champaign, Illinois, and became the president of the Illinois Osteopathic Association. Dr. Astell served on the board of trustees of the Kirksville College of Osteopathic Medicine from 1967 to 1969. She was director of alumni relations and taught in the Department of Osteopathic Methods until 1974.

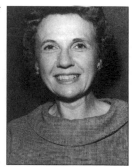

In 1966, she served as president of the Academy of Applied Osteopathy and from 1974 until 1976 she was director of the American Academy of Osteopathy (the organization changed its name in 1970). Among the

Louise Astell, DO
[MOM PH158(25)19]

many honors received by Dr. Astell was an honorary doctor of science in osteopathic medicine from her alma mater in 1975 and the prestigious Andrew Taylor Still Medallion of Honor from the American Academy of Osteopathy in 1977.[59]

Viola Frymann, DO

Viola Frymann was born in England. She graduated from the University of London with a bachelor of medicine/ bachelor of surgery degree and became a member of the Royal College of Surgeons and Licensate of the Royal College of Physicians. She traveled to California to attend the College of Osteopathic Physicians and Surgeons in Los Angeles and received her DO degree in 1949.

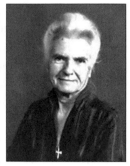

Viola Frymann, DO

For many years Dr. Frymann practiced as a family physician with special emphasis on the diseases of children. In 1982, Dr. Frymann founded the Osteopathic Center for Children, which became a teaching facility of the College of Osteopathic Medicine of the Pacific. The center is involved in the treatment of children, especially those whose primary consideration is prevention of suboptimal health and children with deep and complex problems who seek to reach optimum potential. The Osteopathic Center for Children provides educational courses for DO, MD, and DDS practitioners.

In 1982, Dr. Frymann founded Osteopathy's Promise for Children, a nonprofit organization that funds ongoing research on the unique approach of osteopathic medicine in the treatment of children with severe health problems such as cerebral palsy, seizures, and learning disabilities. Children come from around the world seeking this specialized form of osteopathic medical care. In his introduction to *The Collected Papers of Viola M. Frymann, DO,* Dr. Hollis King wrote:

> The great passion of Dr. Viola Frymann's life has been her work with children. This passion was in part prompted by the loss of her first child and the subsequent realization that osteopathic manipulative medicine, particularly osteopathy in the cranial field, might have prevented this loss. Work with all children, but especially "children with special needs" like cerebral palsy and "learning difficulties," has been the signature characteristics of her work at the Osteopathic Center for Children.[60]

Dr. Viola Frymann is a faculty member at the College of Osteopathic Medicine of the Pacific of the Western University of Health Sciences. She has taught osteopathy at many colleges of osteopathic medicine in the United States as well as at many leading universities throughout the world. She teaches regular courses in France, Italy, and Canada. She has also taught in Switzerland, Belgium, England, China, Japan, Latvia, Russia, Australia, and Denmark.[61]

Dr. Frymann has been a prolific author and researcher, publishing her research on newborn babies, the cranial rhythmic impulse, learning disabilities of children, and the effects of osteopathic manipulative treatment of children with neurological developmental problems, as well as many other medical and osteopathic subjects. She has been the recipient of many awards and honors for her work with children, including the Andrew Taylor Still Medallion of Honor, the highest honor of the American Academy of Osteopathy; the William G. Sutherland Award of the Cranial Academy; Honorary Doctorate of Science in Osteopathic Medicine from the College of Osteopathic Medicine of the Pacific; Osteopathic Physician of the Year from the Osteopathic Physicians and Surgeons of California; the Philip Pumerantz Medal for "distinguished service and extraordinary commitment to the College of Osteopathic Medicine of the Pacific and the osteopathic medical profession" and life membership in Osteopathic Physicians and Surgeons of California for "the sacrifices and labor of love in bringing the osteopathic profession back from extinction." In addition, L'Universite Européenne D'Ostéopathie in Paris named Dr. Viola Frymann docteur honoris causa; the faculty of Le College D'Études Ostéopathiques in Montreal has honored her as their first professeure émérite; and the Centre d'Ostéopathie Atman named her professeure émérite.[62]

Grace H. Kaiser, DO

Grace Kaiser graduated from the Philadelphia College of Osteopathy in 1950.[63] She practiced in rural Lancaster County, Pennsylvania, among the Old Order Amish and Mennonite communities, where she was affectionately known as "Dr. Frau." She was the "baby doctor" to this community, where most of her patients preferred home deliveries and many homes did not have electricity or telephones. For almost three decades and in all kinds of weather, Dr. Frau and her station wagon were a common sight on the back roads of Lancaster County as she traveled to Amish and Mennonite farms to deliver babies. When the snow was too deep and the station wagon could not make it through, she would use

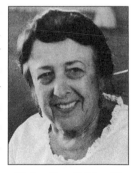

"Dr. Frau," Grace H. Kaiser, DO [Reprinted from *Dr. Frau.* © Good Books (www.GoodBooks.com). Used by permission. All rights reserved.]

a tractor, a sleigh, or even a market wagon to get to her patients. Dr. Frau delivered high-risk patients at the Lancaster Osteopathic Hospital (now the Heart of Lancaster Medical Center), but if there were no complications, mother and baby were discharged four hours after delivery.

At the Lancaster Osteopathic Hospital, Dr. Kaiser taught many interns (including the author!) the fine points of delivering a baby. She was a tough taskmaster who insisted on perfection, a standard that she herself practiced in her daily life.

Dr. Kaiser was loved and respected by her patients. Every year she participated in home deliveries of more babies than most obstetricians deliver in a hospital. This is especially remarkable considering the long distances she traveled to reach her patients. After the deliveries, Dr. Frau would provide medical care for the infants.

In 1978, Dr. Kaiser suffered a tragic accident that left her partially paralyzed and she was forced to retire from medical practice. The Pennsylvania Dutch communities of Lancaster County that she had served with devotion for so many years were devastated by the loss of their beloved Dr. Frau. Even though she could no longer practice medicine, Dr. Kaiser took advantage of forced retirement to write a book about her medical and obstetric practice among the Pennsylvania Dutch communities of Lancaster County. She called her book *Dr. Frau.*[64]

Ruth E. Purdy, DO

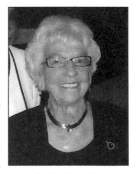

Ruth Purdy worked as an analytical chemist before enrolling in the Philadelphia College of Osteopathy where she earned her DO degree in 1950. She served her internship followed by a residency in internal medicine at Doctors Hospital in Columbus, Ohio, where she was the only female resident physician at that time.

In 1961, Dr. Purdy became the second woman to be accepted as a member of the American College of Internal Medicine; she became a fellow of the American College of Osteopathic Medicine in 1969. In 1963, Dr. Purdy became

Ruth E. Purdy, DO

the director of the first medical intensive care unit in Columbus, located at Doctors Hospital. The unit was so successful that other Columbus hospitals soon patterned their intensive care units after it. She remained director of the ICU until 1975.

Over the years, she served on practically every committee at Doctors Hospital, in addition to serving as president of the staff. Dr. Purdy assisted in the training of medical students from three osteopathic medical colleges and was a faculty member at both the Kirksville and Des Moines Colleges of Osteopathic Medicine.

Dr. Purdy is on the committee for the Hospital Advisory Board, serves as the chair of the New Procedures Committee and is an active member of the senior staff of internists at Doctors Hospital. She is also a member of the board of trustees for both the Central Ohio Heart Association and the Central Ohio Diabetic Association. Dr. Purdy is an active member of the board of trustees for the Philadelphia College of Osteopathic Medicine; she is chair of the Membership Committee and performs multiple other duties. Dr. Purdy has lectured widely and has authored numerous medical articles in the field of internal medicine.[65]

Audrey E. Smith, DO (Lady Audrey E. Percival)

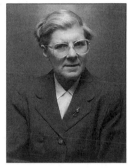

Lady Audrey E. Percival

When Audrey Smith graduated from the British School of Osteopathy in 1951, there were very few women in osteopathy in the United Kingdom. As in the United States, this trend has reversed, and currently about half of all osteopathic students are women.

Upon receiving her DO (diplomate in osteopathy), Dr. Smith went into private practice, which she still maintains today. In addition, she has taught at the British School of Osteopathy. Starting in 1951 as clinical superintendent, she has held numerous positions; in 1967 she was appointed as head of faculty, a position she held until 1986.

From 1965 to 1967, she was president of the Osteopathic Association of Great Britain. From 1967 to 1969, she was a council member of the General Council and Register of Osteopaths and member of the board of directors of the British School of Osteopathy from 1968 until 1986. Dr. Smith prepared the course in osteopathy for the Australian Osteopathic Association for a bachelor of applied science in osteopathy. This course was presented at the Phillip Institute of Technology, Victoria University–Bundoora in Melbourne.

Dr. Smith has published articles in the *British Osteopathic Journal* and contributed five sections of *A Textbook of Osteopathic Diagnosis* (compiled and edited by Peter Hawkins). She has also received multiple awards, including the Littlejohn Award from the Osteopathic Association of Britain, Honorary Life Member of the Australian Osteopathic Association and the British Osteopathic Association, and Honorary Fellow of the British School of Osteopathy.

In 1990, Dr. Smith married Sir Anthony E. Percival; she is now Lady Audrey Percival, although she continues to go by Dr. Smith in her professional life.[66]

Sara Sutton, DO

Sara Sutton graduated from Des Moines Still College of
Osteopathy and Surgery in 1953. She is board certified in
family practice and in neuromusculoskeletal medicine by
the American Academy of Osteopathy.

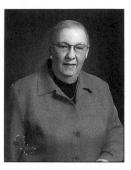

As an intern, Dr. Sutton personally observed how
much more quickly patients recovered with the addition
of osteopathic manipulative techniques, and observed that
selected techniques could increase or decrease the rate of
contractions for patients in labor.

Sara Sutton, DO

For more than fifty years, Dr. Sutton has practiced
osteopathic medicine, usually in private practice as a fam-
ily physician. She has always incorporated osteopathic manipulative techniques
into her practice and has been an outspoken advocate for inclusion of an osteopathic structural examination in routine physical examinations by osteopathic
physicians. She has published articles in the *Journal of the American Osteopathic
Association* on this subject. In addition, Dr. Sutton has been active in the training
of osteopathic medical students, interns, and family practice residents, and was
director of the Family Practice Residency Program at the Des Moines General
Hospital.

Dr. Sutton has received many awards and honors, including Doctor of
Humane Letters from Drake University, the Andrew Taylor Still Medallion of
Honor by the American Academy of Osteopathy, and Physician of the Year by the
Iowa Osteopathic Medical Association. She served as president of the American
Academy of Osteopathy and was also appointed by Iowa Gov. Branstad to the
Respiratory Advisory Committee. She has been an active member of her commu-
nity and has been a member and president of many community organizations. On
top of her active professional and social life, Dr. Sutton still found time to publish
Dr. Sally's Cookbook: With and Without Sin.[67]

Mary L. Butterworth, DO, FAOCA

For more than fifty years, Dr. Butterworth saw incredible advances in the field
of anesthesia and at the Kansas City University of Medicine and Biosciences, in
many cases, she was an integral part of those advances.

Mary Butterworth graduated from the Kansas City College of Osteopathy
and Surgery in 1954.[68] She completed her internship and residency in anesthesiology at the Kansas City College of Osteopathy and Surgery University Hospital

in 1957 and became board certified in anesthesiology in 1968. She was head of the department of anesthesiology at the University Hospital for forty years. She was also medical director of the cardiopulmonary department and director of the pain clinic. Although she served as executive director of the Alumni Association for forty-two years, she considered academic teaching the most pleasurable aspect of her fifty-two-year medical career.

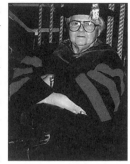

Mary L. Butterworth, DO, FAOCA

For her dedication and lifetime work in osteopathic medicine, Dr. Butterworth received multiple awards from the Missouri Association of Osteopathic Physicians and Surgeons, the American Osteopathic College of Anesthesiologists, and the Kansas City University of Medicine and Biosciences.

Dr. Butterworth was involved in the research and publication of medical articles on the science of anesthesiology and pain management. She established the postanesthesia recovery room, the inhalation therapy department, the pulmonary function laboratory, the cardiac anesthesia program, and the pain management clinic at the Kansas City College of Osteopathy and Surgery University Hospital. She also instituted medical student rotation through the anesthesia department at the hospital.[69]

Isabelle A. Chapello, DO

After receiving her bachelor's degree from Rockford College and her master's degree from the University of Wisconsin, Isabelle Chapello attended the Chicago College of Osteopathic Medicine, earning her DO degree in 1955. She was certified by the American Board of Family Practice in 1976 and was also certified in osteopathic manipulative medicine in 1979. She maintains special proficiency in cranial osteopathic manipulation. Dr. Chapello traveled to Nanjing, China, where she studied *Tui na*, an ancient Chinese form of medicine and massage dating back to the Shang Dynasty, circa 1700 BCE. She was certified in *Tui na* by the World Health Organization in 1987.

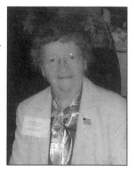

Isabelle A. Chapello, DO, FAAO

After completing her internship at the Parkview Osteopathic Hospital, Dr. Chapello established a family practice in Luna Pier, Michigan, in 1956. Even now, over fifty years later, she still maintains that practice. She had active hospital privileges at the Parkview Osteopathic Hospital from 1956 until the hospital closed in 1994.

Dr. Chapello also used her medical expertise in her community. She was Monroe County's first chief deputy medical examiner and interim chief medical examiner. She was also a nursing home evaluator and worked with the Monroe County Migrant Clinics and Polio Vaccine Clinics. In addition, she has worked with the Monroe County Red Cross Blood Bank for over ten years and with the Michigan Association of Community Mental Health Services Boards and Department of Mental Health. Dr. Chapello has also published articles in the *American Association of Osteopathy Journal* and in the *National Woman's Health Report*.[70]

Eleanor Masterson, DO

Eleanor Masterson graduated from New York University before attending the Philadelphia College of Osteopathy, where she also served her internship. She received her DO in 1957.

Dr. Masterson was an instructor at the college clinics for several years. In 1968, she was named director of the Philadelphia College of Osteopathic Medicine clinics; she was the first female to be named director and held that position until 1978. While director she started new specialty clinics, such as endocrinology and proctology, and improved the management of the clinics through a protocol of procedures that included an improved scheduling system. She also initiated the protocol requiring osteo-

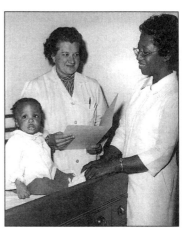

Eleanor Masterson, DO (left)
with head nurse
[1957 *Synapsis*, PCOM]

pathic medical students to visit their clinic patients who were admitted to the hospital and to be present during their patient's surgical procedures, thus creating the dual benefit of teaching the student continuity of care as well as providing reassurance for the patients. Dr. Masterson also initiated the clinic Christmas party that included giving gifts for the children who attended the clinics.[71]

Eileen L. DiGiovanna, DO, FAAO

Eileen DiGiovanna graduated from the Chicago College of Osteopathic Medicine in 1959. She is board certified in neuromusculoskeletal medicine, osteopathic manipulative medicine, family practice, pain management, and forensic medicine.

Many modern osteopathic physicians have studied manipulative techniques using her textbook, *An Osteopathic Approach to Diagnosis and Treatment*. This book, now in its third edition, is the standard textbook on osteopathic manipulation and is used by many osteopathic medical schools, so that students frequently refer to "studying from DiGiovanna."[72]

In 2002, Dr. DiGiovanna authored *An Encyclopedia of Osteopathy* and coauthored two chapters in *Foundations for Osteopathic Medicine*.[73] She has been on the editorial board of the *Journal of the American Osteopathic Association* and the publications committee of the American Academy of Osteopathy. In addition, she has done research on the force generated during osteopathic manipulative treatments, and has published and spoken widely on the many aspects of osteopathic medicine.

Dr. DiGiovanna started her teaching career as an assistant professor of osteopathic manipulative medicine at the New York College of Osteopathic Medicine in 1977 and has held many positions at that college. She was the associate dean for Student Affairs and now serves as associate dean emerita.[74]

Ethel Allen, DO

The Dr. Ethel Allen Elementary School in North Philadelphia stands as a symbol of the achievements of the short but energetic and praiseworthy career of Dr. Ethel Allen. Ethel Allen graduated from Hallahan Catholic High School for Girls in central Philadelphia and from West Virginia State College with majors in chemistry and biology and a minor in mathematics. In spite of her good undergraduate grades and high scores on the Medical College Admissions Test, Allen was repeatedly denied admission to medical school. In a 1978 interview, she told a *Philadelphia Inquirer* reporter, "for seven years I was discriminated against for being black and female."[75] She was finally accepted at the

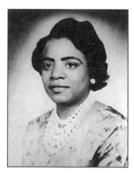

"Ghetto Doctor" Ethel Allen, DO
[1963 *Synapsis*, PCOM]

Philadelphia College of Osteopathy where she received her DO degree in 1963; she completed her internship in Michigan. True to her roots, she returned to establish her medical practice in North Philadelphia, where she proudly referred to herself as a "GD," or "Ghetto Doctor," and listed her specialty as "Ghetto Medicine."[76] She became medical director of the Model Cities Program for the City of Philadelphia.

Dr. Allen never had any intention of going into politics, but the conditions she encountered in the North Philadelphia ghettos pulled her in that direction. In her first campaign, she ran as a Republican for Philadelphia City Council in 1971, and was widely considered to have no chance of winning a seat on the overwhelmingly Democratic council. In her one debate against the popular three-term Democratic incumbent, Dr. Allen spoke first. She said, "In the interest of brevity, let me just say that I am a candidate. Whatever my opponent hasn't done, I will do. Whatever he has done, I will do better," and then promptly sat down. Her opponent rose to reply, sputtered, and then sat down as well. Dr. Allen won the election handily.[77]

Dr. Allen soon earned the reputation of a feisty politician, winning reelection to the city council in 1975. Shortly after her reelection, the mayor of Philadelphia took what Dr. Allen regarded as the wrong stand on a controversial housing project for minorities. Dr. Allen warned him in a fiery speech that *"una scupa nuava*—a new broom sweeps clean." She added, "If you push me, I may have to run against you, Mr. Mayor. And when I run, I win."[78]

As Philadelphia's first black councilwoman, much of Dr. Allen's efforts focused on reducing gang violence. The number of gang-related deaths in Philadelphia when she was elected was seventy-five per year; by 1977 this figure had dropped to zero.[79]

Dr. Allen maintained her practice of ghetto medicine three nights a week while serving on the Philadelphia City Council. She also served on the boards of the YMCA, United Way, and the NAACP. She was a member of the National Black Elected Officials Organization, the Black Women's Political Caucus, and the National Women's Political Caucus. She was the chairperson of the Ford for President Committee, and it was Dr. Allen who seconded Gerald Ford's nomination for president of the United States at the Republican National Convention. During her life she received many awards, including the prestigious Gimbel Philadelphia Award. Dr. Allen frequently stated that she represented four minorities—she was a woman, a black, an osteopathic physician, and a Republican on the Philadelphia City Council.[80]

In 1978, the governor-elect appointed Dr. Allen to the position of secretary of the Commonwealth of Pennsylvania. When she accepted this position, she became the highest-ranking black woman state official in the nation. She was also the first woman, the first black, and the first osteopathic physician to be named to this high position. Dr. Allen was an up-and-coming politician. She refused the Republican Party's request to run for a seat in the US Congress because she was seriously being considered as a candidate for mayor of Philadelphia, a position it was widely believed she could have easily won.[81] There was speculation that Dr. Allen would become a frontrunner in state and national politics. This speculation, however, ended when she was diagnosed with breast cancer, a battle she was on the way to winning when she was diagnosed with advanced heart disease. Dr. Allen's promising career was cut short when she died in 1981 from heart disease at fifty-two years of age.[82]

In 1982, a Philadelphia women's group recognized Dr. Allen by commissioning a bas-relief to honor her not only for her contributions to medicine and politics, but also for her contributions to women's rights. The bas-relief was displayed in the Afro-American Historical and Cultural Museum in Philadelphia before being moved to the Dr. Ethel Allen Elementary School.[83]

NOTES

1. Hildreth, *Lengthening Shadow of Dr. Andrew Taylor Still*, 204–8.

2. "From President Willard: Materia Medica," *JAOA* 25 (Dec. 1925): 279–80.

3. "Proceedings of the House of Delegates," *Forum of Osteopathy* 3 (Aug. 1929): supp. 5–8.

4. "Nature of Osteopathy," *JAMA* 89 (Oct. 1927): 1354–55.

5. McCole, "Osteopathic Definitions," *Forum of Osteopathy* 10 (1936): 151–68.

6. Gevitz, *The DOs*, 95.

7. "Entrance Requirements, Next Steps," *JAOA* 39 (1939): 225–26.

8. Gevitz, *The DOs*, 96.

9. Riley, "Osteopathy's First Half Century," *JAOA* 23 (July 1924): 821–22.

10. Gevitz, *The DOs*, 94.

11. Jones, *Difference a DO Makes*, 35.

12. Ibid., 35.

13. The initial law providing for the commissioning of DOs as medical officers was passed in 1917 (HR 5407). Congress again provided for the commissioning of osteopathic physicians in the armed services in 1941 (Pub. L. No. 139, 55 Stat. 300 [1941]) and 1942 (Pub. L. No. 763, Military Appropriations Act, 55 Stat. 366 [1942]).

14. Gevitz, *The DOs*, 98.

15. Jones, *Difference a DO Makes*, 34–35.

16. Walter, *Women and Osteopathic Medicine*, 21.

17. Gevitz, *The DOs*, 96.

18. Jane Denslow, Kathleen Eubanks, and Jeff White, "American Schools of Osteopathic Medicine, 1892–2007," MOM; and Willard, "Where Our Students Come From," *JAOA* 46 (1947): 313.

19. Gevitz *The DOs*, 96.

20. Mills, "Applications to Osteopathic Colleges," *JAOA* 51, no. 6 (1952): 541–42.

21. "Important Change in Hospital Construction Act Regulations," *JAOA* 46 (1947): 570.

22. Miller, *A Second Voice*, 52–53.

23. Perloff, *To Secure Merit*, 39.

24. Walsh, *Doctors Wanted: No Women Need Apply*, 179; and Mills, "Doctors Wanted: Women Urged to Apply," *Forum of Osteopathy* 20 (Dec. 1946): 289–97.

25. Gevitz, *The DOs*, 45; and Armstrong and Armstrong, *Great American Medicine Show*, 45.

26. Jones, *Difference a DO Makes*, 29, 35, 45–49.

27. *Metropolitan University, College of Medicine and Surgery, Graduate Division, Annual Catalogue* (Los Angeles, 1945); Metropolitan University file, microfilm, AOA Archives, Chicago; and "Minutes of the American Osteopathic Association Board of Trustees, July 1946," 171–75, microfilm, AOA Archives, Chicago.

28. "Report of the American Osteopathic Association Conference Committee to the AOA House of Delegates, July 1954," microfilm, AOA Archives, Chicago; "Supplemental Report of the Board of Trustees," *JAMA* 156 (1954): 1600–1605; "Report of the Committee for the Study of Relations between Osteopathy and Medicine," *JAMA* 158 (1955):736–42.

29. "Minutes of the Meeting of the American Osteopathic Association Conference Committee, June 11, 1955," microfilm, AOA Archives, Chicago, 1–5; and Gevitz, *The DOs,* 126–27.

30. Carpenter, "More Women Needed," Letters to the AOA, *Forum of Osteopathy* (Apr. 1953): 5.

31. "Osteopathic vs. Medical Hospital Efficiency," *JAOA* 32, no. 4 (1932): 133–35.

32. "Osteopathic Unit Makes Excellent Showing in Annual Report," *Western Osteopath* 24 (Sept. 1929): 7–10.

33. Armenta, "Unit 2: Osteopathic Medicine's Experiment at Los Angeles County General Hospital," *The DO* 50, no. 5 (2009): 44.

34. "Osteopathic vs. Medical Hospital Efficiency," *JAOA* 32, no. 4 (1932): 133–35.

35. Getitz, *The DOs,* 116.

36. Armenta, "Unit 2: Osteopathic Medicine's Experiment at Los Angeles County General Hospital," *The DO* 50, no. 5 (2009): 44.

37. Rogers, "Report of the Bureau of Professional Education and Colleges," *JAOA* 36 (1937): 607.

38. "Proceedings of the House of Delegates," *JAOA* 40 (1940): 33–34.

39. Gevitz, *The DOs,* 115–19.

40. "MDs Can Teach DOs—If," *AOA News Bulletin* 3 (June 1959): 1–2.

41. "Report of the Judicial Council," *JAMA* 171 (1959): 978–79.

42. "Text of Michigan Resolution," *AOA News Bulletin* 3 (Aug. 1959): 1.

43. Bartosh, "History of Osteopathy in California," *Journal of the Osteopathic Physicians and Surgeons of California* 5 (Apr.–May 1978): 30–33.

44. "Osteopathy: Special Report of the Judicial Council to the AMA House of Delegates," *JAMA* 177 (1961): 775.

45. "Text of Michigan Resolution," *AOA News Bulletin* 3 (Aug. 1959): 3; "COA Charter Revoked," *AOA News Bulletin* 3 (Nov. 1960): 1; and "AOA Charters New Group," *AOA News Bulletin* 4 (Feb. 1961): 1.

46. Gevitz, *The DOs,* 133–34. The college is now known as the University of California College of Medicine, Irvine.

47. "Chronology of Capitulation," *The DO* (Sept. 1961): 35.

48. Multiple editorials in the *JAOA* written by George Northup; and DiGiovanna, *Encyclopedia of Osteopathy,* 69.

49. Gevitz, *The DOs,* 133–34.

50. "Pennsylvania DOs Back AOA Policies," *Journal of the POMA* 5, no. 3 (Summer 1963): 8.

51. "Washington State MD-DO Plan Told," *AMA News* 6 (11 Nov. 1963): 16.

52. Gevitz, *The DOs,* 133.

53. Leahy, "How DOs Feel about AOA-AMA Relations," *Osteopathic Physician* 38 (July 1972): 28.

54. Gevitz, *The DOs*, 139; and Kisch and Viseltear, *Doctors of Medicine and Doctors of Osteopathy in California*, 41–42.

55. "A Period of Uncertainty," 28; "Profile of a Merger: Responses to Questionnaires, Analyses, Comments Conducted 17–20 November 1965, in California by the AOA Public Relations Department," microfilm, AOA Archives, Chicago; and Leahy, "How DOs Feel about AOA-AMA Relations," *Osteopathic Physician* 38 (July 1972): 28.

56. AOA Fact Sheet, 1965.

57. Perloff, *To Secure Merit*, 49.

58. DiGiovanna, *Encyclopedia of Osteopathy*, 47.

59. Ibid., 15–16.

60. King, *Collected Papers of Viola M. Frymann*, ix.

61. Osteopathic Center for Children, "Helping All Children Reach Their Potential since 1982," accessed 15 Oct. 2006, www.osteopathiccenter.org/bios.html, .

62. Osteopathic Center for Children, "Osteopathy's Promise to Children," accessed 11 Oct. 2006, www.osteopathiccenter.org/promise.html.

63. *PCOM 1999 Alumni Directory, Centennial Edition*, 67.

64. Dr. Grace Kaiser and the author were friends and professional associates for many years in Lancaster County, Pennsylvania.

65. Ruth Purdy, personal correspondence with the author, 3 January 2007.

66. Lady Audrey Percival, personal correspondence with the author, 1 January 2007.

67. Sara Sutton, personal correspondence with the author, 10 February 2007.

68. In 1970 Kansas City College Osteopathy and Surgery became the Kansas City College of Osteopathic Medicine. Ten years later, the school's name was changed to the University of Health Sciences. Finally, in 2004, the institution was renamed the Kansas City University of Medicine and Biosciences.

69. Mary Butterworth, personal correspondence with the author, 28 January 2007.

70. Isabelle Chappello, personal correspondence with the author, 25 January 2007.

71. Perloff, *To Secure Merit*, 85.

72. DiGiovanna, Schiowitz, and Dowling, *An Osteopathic Approach to Diagnosis and Treatment*, 3rd ed.

73. Ward, *Foundations for Osteopathic Medicine*, 2nd ed. 1017-25; 1143-52.

74. Eileen DiGiovanna, personal correspondence with the author, 5 December 2006.

75. Jack Severson, "Despite Her New Post, Does Mayoralty Still Beckon?" *Philadelphia Inquirer*, 16 August 1978.

76. "Ex-Thornburgh Aide Dies in Philadelphia," *Towanda Daily Review*, 17 December 1981.

77. Obituary, *Philadelphia Bulletin*, 17 December 1981.

78. Jane Eisner, "For Life of Achievement, Dr. Allen Receives Recognition in Bronze," *Philadelphia Inquirer*, 17 December 1982.

79. "Allan Brings Record of Service," *Philadelphia Bulletin*, 3 January 1979.

80. Burr Van Atta, "Ethel Allen Dies; Was on City Council," *Philadelphia Inquirer*, 17 December 1981.

81. Jack Severson, "Despite Her New Post, Does Mayoralty Still Beckon?" *Philadelphia Inquirer*, 16 August 1978.

82. "Ex-Thornburgh Aide Dies in Philadelphia," *Towanda Daily Review*, 17 December 1981.

83. Jane Eisner, "For Life of Achievement, Dr. Allen Receives Recognition in Bronze," *Philadelphia Inquirer*, 17 December 1982.

Chapter Five

The Modern Era of Osteopathic Medicine, 1965 to Present

"The most any physician can do for a patient is to render operative the forces within the body itself."

Andrew Taylor Still, MD, DO

"The feet of women are marching towards medicine, and there's no way we cannot break through doors—just because of sheer numbers."

Geraldine T. O'Shea, DO

IN 1964, THE FIVE REMAINING OSTEOPATHIC MEDICAL SCHOOLS graduated only four female DOs, a meager 1.1 percent of the combined graduating class of all five schools. In that year, there were only twenty-three women enrolled in the osteopathic medical schools, representing only 1.8 percent of the combined student body. The osteopathic profession started to recover its female enrollment rate beginning in 1965, two years before the allopathic female enrollment rate began to recover.[1] Thus 1965 can be seen as the beginning of the modern era for women in osteopathic medicine.

In 1969, the colleges of osteopathic medicine had a combined female student enrollment rate of 3 percent, and female enrollment continued to increase in the succeeding years. However, during this same period, the number of women entering allopathic medical schools increased even more. In 1969, the MD schools had a 9 percent female enrollment rate and by 1993 40.2 percent of all students enrolling were women. This is the only period when allopathic schools had a higher percentage of women enrolling than osteopathic schools. By 1988, the MD schools already had an enrollment of 35 percent women, and it took the DO schools five years to catch up. The exact reason for this discrepancy in female enrollment remains unclear, but it appears that there were not as many female applicants to the osteopathic schools. In October 1995, the *Journal of the American Osteopathic*

Association printed an article calling for the recruiting of more female applicants to osteopathic colleges.[2]

Nearly fifty years had passed since the A. T. Still College of Osteopathy and Surgery opened in 1922 and merged with the American School of Osteopathy two years later. That was the last new osteopathic college for a long time. In the years between, osteopathic colleges either closed or merged, but no new schools opened. There was no continuous expansion of the profession, only the fluctuations caused by the increase in entrance requirements, economics, and war. After the loss of an osteopathic college and over two thousand DOs in California in the late 1960s, the profession, more than ever before, needed to grow.[3]

Percentage of female students in osteopathic medical colleges	
1973	6.5
1978	16.3
1980	19.7
1985	27.7
1990	32.7
1995	36.3
2000	41.1
2005	49.6
2007	50.0

SOURCE: AOA, *Osteopathic Medical Profession Report*, 2008, 7–8.

At the same time, the osteopathic profession continued to fight the efforts of the American Medical Association (AMA) to convert the remaining osteopathic medical schools into allopathic medical schools. After successfully defeating the eclectic medical profession in the 1930s and the homeopathic medical profession in the 1950s, the AMA was frustrated by their failure to eliminate the osteopathic medical profession during the 1960s. Determined to preserve the doctrine that "there cannot be two distinct sciences of medicine or two different yet equally valid systems of medical practice,"[4] the AMA in July 1967 authorized its board to begin negotiations with the five remaining osteopathic medical schools for the purpose of converting them into allopathic medical schools. Only the economically weak Des Moines College of Osteopathy and Surgery agreed to meet with representatives of the AMA, but negotiations broke down after the school's administration was replaced with DOs loyal to the profession. In 1968, the AMA changed tactics, asking each of its county and state medical organizations to accept DOs and encouraging the opening of allopathic residency training programs to osteopathic physicians so that DOs could sit for allopathic board certification examinations.[5] This may have sounded like a positive move to DOs who had struggled for recognition, but it was just another, although perhaps better disguised, attempt to absorb the osteopathic medical profession into the allopathic medical profession.

In the meantime, in 1966 the Michigan State Senate had voted to establish the first state-supported osteopathic college of medicine. However, when the measure was brought up for consideration by the full house in 1967, the Michigan State Medical Society organized strong opposition to the bill and managed to have to have it defeated by a scant two votes. It would be another two years before osteopaths were able to have the bill brought back to the state legislature. In the meantime, the board of trustees of the school decided to open the school without state funding. The school inducted its first class in 1969, becoming the first new osteopathic school in forty-seven years. When the bill came before the Michigan legislature for the second time, the osteopathic advocates were better organized, and the bill passed and was signed into law by the governor. With state funding, the new osteopathic medical school was incorporated into Michigan State University and transferred from Pontiac to East Lansing, where its infrastructure was provided by the university. The reestablished college was called Michigan State University, College of Osteopathic Medicine. Michigan State University already had an allopathic medical school—the College of Human Medicine, which shared with the new osteopathic college the same pool of basic science professors. There were some separate classes for DO and MD students;[6] however, the very fact that the osteopathic and allopathic medical schools were side by side on the same university campus served as visible evidence that the two American medical professions and philosophies were indeed separate but equal.[7]

The late 1960s also saw the first DOs to be commissioned as medical officers in the military. Despite several laws being passed to allow the commissioning of osteopathic physicians as medical officers, the allopathic medicine profession had created barriers to prevent any DOs from actually being commissioned. Finally, in 1967, the first group of DOs were commissioned. None of the initial 111 osteopathic physicians were women however, since at that time men dominated the profession. For more on osteopathic physicians in the military, see chapter 7.

In the fall of 1970, a private osteopathic college opened in Fort Worth, Texas. Initially housed in the top two floors of the Fort Worth Osteopathic Hospital, the new school spent its first year eagerly waiting to establish itself as a state-funded medical college in a region that was new to osteopathic medical education. In 1971, the school received initial limited state funding, and in 1973 this funding was significantly increased. In 1975, the Texas College of Osteopathic Medicine was established as a public institution under the Board of Regents of the North Texas State University. The osteopathic profession now had two medical schools affiliated with universities and supported by public funds.[8] The establishment of these two new osteopathic medical schools ushered in the greatest period of growth and expansion in the profession's history, and also marked the true beginning of government funding and university affiliations, two areas that had previously made osteopathic education vulnerable to forces hostile to the profession.

The 1970s saw tumultuous changes in American society and politics, and the osteopathic profession was not without its own transformation. A critical factor to this new expansion and change was the outstanding performance of osteopathic medical students in standardized testing. In 1970, there were thirteen states that required DO graduates to pass the identical examination taken by the MD graduates, providing an opportunity to compare DO and MD graduates. The medical licensing statistics, published in the *Journal of the AMA*, showed that the failure rate for the licensure examination by American osteopathic graduates was only 1.5 percent, compared to failure rates of 9.3 percent for American medical graduates, 14.0 percent for Canadian medical graduates, and 37.3 percent for international medical graduates.[9] These statistics provided the strongest argument yet against the allegation that osteopathic education was somehow inferior to allopathic education.

In 1973, Mississippi, which had no practicing osteopathic physicians at the time, became the last state to grant full, unlimited practice rights to DOs.[10] In 1974, new osteopathic colleges opened in Oklahoma and West Virginia;[11] both became state-supported medical schools. As the osteopathic medical education community continued to establish reputable and quality programs throughout the nation, adding to the prestige of osteopathic medical philosophy and tradition, the merger fight in California continued its bitter dispute on to the California Supreme Court. Finally, in 1974, the court, in a unanimous decision, declared unconstitutional the 1962 legislation forbidding the licensing of new DOs in California.[12] Since that ruling, two new osteopathic medical schools have opened in California: the Western University College of Osteopathic Medicine in Pomona (1977) and the Touro College of Osteopathic Medicine in Vallejo (1997).

The unregulated growth of unauthorized schools and diploma mills that plagued the early years of the profession played no role in this new period of expansion and may have even provided the original impetus to improve the vigorous quality and accreditation standards now in place. Each of these new modern osteopathic medical colleges is inspected and regulated by the American Osteopathic Association and the American Association of Colleges of Osteopathic Medicine. As of January 2011, there are thirty functioning osteopathic medical colleges in the United States, with still more colleges in the process of development.

OSTEOPATHIC MEDICAL COLLEGES: year established, current name, and location

1892   A. T. Still University–Kirksville College of Osteopathic Medicine (Kirksville, Missouri)

1898   Des Moines University–College of Osteopathic Medicine (Des Moines, Iowa)

1899   Philadelphia College of Osteopathic Medicine (Philadelphia, Pennsylvania)

1900   Midwestern University–Chicago College of Osteopathic Medicine (Chicago, Illinois)

1916   Kansas City University of Medicine and Bioscience–College of Osteopathic Medicine (Kansas City, Missouri)

1969   Michigan State University–College of Osteopathic Medicine (East Lansing, Michigan)

1970   University of North Texas Health Sciences Center–Texas College of Osteopathic Medicine (Fort Worth, Texas)

1972   Oklahoma State University Center for Health Sciences–College of Osteopathic Medicine (Tulsa, Oklahoma)

       West Virginia School of Osteopathic Medicine (Lewisburg, West Virginia)

       New York College of Osteopathic Medicine of the New York Institute of Technology (Old Westbury, New York)

1975   Ohio University–College of Osteopathic Medicine (Athens, Ohio)

1976   University of Medicine and Dentistry of New Jersey–School of Osteopathic Medicine (Stratford, New Jersey)

1977   Western University of Health Sciences–College of Osteopathic Medicine of the Pacific (Pamona, California)

1978   University of New England–College of Osteopathic Medicine (Biddeford, Maine)

1979   Nova Southeastern University–College of Osteopathic Medicine (Fort Lauderdale, Florida)

1992   Lake Erie College of Osteopathic Medicine (Erie, Pennsylvania)

1995   Midwestern University–Arizona College of Osteopathic Medicine (Glendale, Arizona)

1997   Pikesville College School of Osteopathic Medicine (Pikesville, Kentucky)

       Touro University College of Osteopathic Medicine–California (Vallejo, California)

2003   Edward Via Virginia College of Osteopathic Medicine (Blacksburg, Virginia)

2004   Lake Erie College of Osteopathic Medicine–Bradenton (Bradenton, Florida)

       Touro University–Nevada College of Osteopathic Medicine (Henderson, Nevada)

       Philadelphia College of Osteopathic Medicine–Georgia Campus (Suwanee, Georgia)

2005   Pacific Northwest University of Health Sciences College of Osteopathic Medicine (Yakima, Washington)

2006   Lincoln Memorial University DeBusk College of Osteopathic Medicine (Harrogate, Tennessee)

       Touro College of Osteopathic Medicine (New York City, New York)

       Rocky Vista College of Osteopathic Medicine (Aurora, Colorado)

2007   A. T. Still University School of Osteopathic Medicine in Arizona (Mesa, Arizona)

2008   William Carey University College of Osteopathic Medicine (Hattiesburg, Mississippi)

2010   Via Virginia College of Osteopathic Medicine–Spartanburg (Spartanburg, South Carolina)

2012*   Marian University College of Osteopathic Medicine (Indianapolis, Indiana)

       Alabama College of Osteopathic Medicine (Dolthan, Alabama)

*Projected date

The rapid growth of the profession as a whole was matched with the steady growth of female enrollment. In 1969, only 2.4 percent of the first-year classes were female, while thirty-four years later, in 2003, women entering osteopathic medical schools outnumbered the male students. Since then, female enrollment has remained close to 50 percent.[13] Public acceptance of the osteopathic profession is higher now than ever before. Measured by a national survey, patients of osteopathic physicians reported the highest levels of satisfaction when compared to patients of other physician and nonphysician practitioners.[14] Today, osteopathic physicians provide over sixty million patient visits yearly and offer high-quality health care to the American people alongside their allopathic counterparts, while using differing but complimentary philosophies.[15]

A study published by the US Department of Health, Education, and Welfare in 1976 compared the costs of education for seven health care professions. This study showed that the cost of medical professional education was highest for osteopathic medicine, followed by dentistry, allopathic medicine, podiatry, optometry, veterinary medicine, and pharmacy (the least expensive). This study also showed that osteopathic medical students received the smallest average scholarships and had the greatest percentage of students taking out educational loans. The average debt of an osteopathic medical student was 30 percent greater than the average debt of dental students, the group ranking second highest in debt load. One of the most obvious reasons that osteopathic education was the most expensive in 1976 was that the osteopathic profession received far less in government subsidies than the other professions. This situation, although still far from being equal, has shown steady improvement over the years. Almost all of the women who responded to the 1976 survey spoke about problems they encountered in financing their osteopathic education. The study states that, "Both male and female respondents recognized that problems with financial support affected women differently than men, and female students believed that men have an easier time getting loans and getting support from their families."[16]

In recent decades, there have also been studies of gender-related trends in medicine. Female physicians trend toward pediatrics, internal medicine, family practice, psychiatry, and obstetrics-gynecology, which have traditionally been the lower-paid specialties. Male physicians, DOs and MDs alike, tend to predominate in the higher-paid areas of specialization. Other trends are the tendency for female physicians to prefer office-based practice over hospital-based practice, and the higher likelihood of female, rather than male, physicians to work for a salary.[17] In addition to, or perhaps even in spite of these trends, there are some female physicians who have obtained high academic positions, serving as deans and provosts in colleges of osteopathic medicine.

The trend toward ever-increasing numbers of female medical students has inevitably led to changes in many training programs. Frequently, accommodations must be made for women who are pregnant or who have the responsibility of caring for young children. Not all schools or faculties agree with the practice of giving accommodation to one person with a special need while insisting that everyone is treated equally. A study of the women who graduated from Yale University School of Medicine between 1922 and 1999 showed that 82 percent of the women physicians over forty years of age had become mothers. This same study showed that most of the female physicians who did not have children had specialized in one of the surgical fields. Of the women who had graduated before 1950, only 24 percent gave birth to children while they were in medical school. Between 1950 and 1989, a full 42 percent of the women had children during their medical training. The average age of women entering medical school varied. In the 1950s, 95.7 percent of female medical students were under twenty-four years old, but in the 1990s, 34.5 percent of women were twenty-four or older when they entered medical school.[18]

Once in practice, many female physicians are faced with the reality that a demanding medical career will conflict with their need to be available for children and family responsibilities. Some women may choose specialties with relatively set hours and little or no after-hour calls such as pathology or emergency medicine. Others may choose to join large groups where night and weekend coverage is shared by many physicians. Working as a salaried physician in a clinic or hospital will appeal to others. It is likely that many of the practices adopted by large employers, such as job sharing and flexible hours, will become common in the medical practice of the future.

More and more advertisements for physicians in medical journals are offering part-time, flexible hours, no hospital rounds, and little or no on-call requirements. In 2007, 19 percent of physicians worked only part-time and that number is rising yearly. Nearly two-thirds of all part-time physicians are women between the ages of thirty and fifty. The remaining one-third are men over sixty.[19] There are presently few women physicians in the over-sixty age group, but this is expected to change in the future.

The National Osteopathic Women Physicians Association was established in 1989 and Isabelle Chapello, DO, was elected its first president. The association is an outgrowth of the woman's organization Delta Omega, founded in 1904 by eight female osteopathic students at the American School of Osteopathy. The Greek letters *delta omega* were chosen to represent "DO."[20]

WOMEN GRADUATING BETWEEN 1965 AND THE PRESENT
Pauline M. Schultz, DO

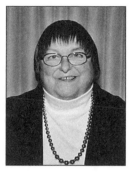

After graduating from the University of Pennsylvania with a major in chemistry, Pauline M. Delia Schultz received her DO degree from the Philadelphia College of Osteopathy in 1966, the only female member of her graduating class. Dr. Schultz practiced osteopathic medicine for thirty-seven years in the Philadelphia and New Jersey areas and retired in 2004. She maintained close organizational ties with the osteopathic profession during the course of her professional career, and practiced full-time even while raising her children. While her children were young, Dr. Schultz arranged her professional schedule in

Pauline M. Schultz, DO

order to work nights in the emergency department and also as a house medical officer at the Zurbrugg Memorial Hospital in Riverside, New Jersey, when her husband, Harry Schultz, could be home with their children. This allowed her to take her children to school, act as a homeroom mother, and serve on the Parent Teacher Association as well. Looking back, Dr. Schultz states, "Achieving this balance between a career and home life is a difficult challenge, which many female physicians struggle with."[21]

Alison A. Clarey, DO

Alison A. Clarey graduated from the College of Osteopathic Medicine and Surgery at Des Moines University in 1972 and completed her internship and residency in general surgery at the Grandview Hospital in Dayton, Ohio, in 1977. She was board certified in general surgery in 1982, the only female osteopathic physician certified in general surgery that year. She has been a member of the American College of Osteopathic Surgeons since 1981 and became a fellow of that specialty college in 1987.

Dr. Clarey has had a successful general surgical practice in Dayton since 1978. She is the program director in general surgery at Grandview Hospital and a clinical professor of general surgery at Wright State University Medical School. She is a member of the medical advisory board at Ohio University College of

Osteopathic Medicine in Athens, Ohio, and served as chief of staff at Grandview and Southview Hospitals in 1991 and 1992.

Dr. Clarey has been recognized for her work in providing free surgical care for indigent patients and for assisting with service projects to local organizations in the Dayton area. She does not limit her charitable works to her local area, working around the world as a volunteer with the Society Taking Active Responsibility for International Self Help (STARFISH). Dr. Clarey has provided humanitarian surgical care to the medically underserved countries of Sierra Leone, Madagascar, and Guatemala. On 15 September 2006, Dr. Clarey became the first female surgeon to become president of the American College of Osteopathic Surgeons. Dr. Clarey is an accomplished pilot and belongs to several pilot associations.[22]

Barbara Ross-Lee, DO

Barbara Ross-Lee graduated from the Michigan State University, College of Osteopathic Medicine in 1973. She ran a solo family practice in Detroit before turning to teaching medicine. A fellow of the American Board of Family Physicians, Dr. Ross-Lee has lectured widely and published numerous scholarly articles on a variety of medical and health care issues. She served as chair of the department of family medicine and associate dean for health policy at Michigan State University, College of Osteopathic Medicine.

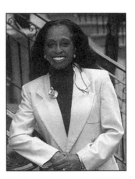

Barbara Ross-Lee, DO, FACOPP

Dr. Ross-Lee has been CEO of Academic Health Centers and president of Faculty Practice Plan since 2001, and served as dean of Michigan State University, College of Osteopathic Medicine from 1993 to 2001, the first African American woman to be appointed dean of an American medical school. She has an extensive background in health policy issues and serves as an advisor on primary care, medical education, minority health, women's health, and rural health care issues on the federal and state levels.

Dr. Ross-Lee is executive director of the National Osteopathic Center for Health Policy. She serves as director of training in policy studies for postgraduate osteopathic trainees (resident physicians), as director of the Institute for National Health Policy and Research, and executive director of the National Osteopathic Medical Association. These are but a few of her many accomplishments along with numerous awards, which include being inducted into The Ohio Women's Hall of Fame in 1998 and receiving the 2003 Dale Dodson

Award from the American Association of Colleges of Osteopathic Medicine for outstanding leadership in osteopathic medicine.[23]

Virginia A. Syperda, DO

Virginia Syperda graduated from the Chicago College of Osteopathic Medicine in 1975. She is married to classmate Glenn Syperda, DO, who is an anesthesiologist. After serving a rotating internship at the Lansing General Hospital, Dr. Syperda went into general practice in Lansing, Michigan, from 1976 until 1982. She was the chairperson of general practice and director of outpatient services at Provincial Hospital from 1977 to 1979. She served as cochairperson of the general practice department at Lansing General Hospital from 1980 to 1982.

After obtaining experience in general practice, Dr. Syperda served her residency in diagnostic radiology from 1982 through 1985 at Flint Osteopathic Hospital. She was certified in diagnostic radiology in 1986 by the American Osteopathic Board of Radiology and served as a staff radiologist at several hospitals and out-patient facilities, including the US Air Force PRIMUS clinic in Brandon, Florida.

Dr. Syperda received her MBA degree from the University of South Florida in 1993 and her doctor of education degree from the Nova Southeastern University in Florida in 2001. She was a professor of radiology at the Lake Erie College of Osteopathic Medicine, Bradenton, where she was the principal investigator for a radiology-based research project. Dr. Syperda is presently a professor of radiology and primary care, as well as the director of physical diagnosis at Lake Erie College of Osteopathic Medicine Seton Hill in Greensberg, Pennsylvania.[24]

Silvia M. Ferretti, DO

Silvia Ferretti graduated from the Philadelphia College of Osteopathic Medicine in 1977 and served her internship at the college hospital. She served her residency in physical medicine and rehabilitation at the Hospital of the University of Pennsylvania where she was an assistant clinical professor of physical medicine and rehabilitation from 1982 to 1984. Dr. Ferretti was a professor and chairperson of the department of physical medicine and rehabilitation of Philadelphia College of Osteopathic Medicine from 1984 to 1987. She is board certified in physical medicine and rehabilitation, family practice, and geriatric medicine.

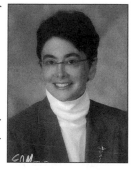

Silvia M. Ferretti, DO

Dr. Ferretti is chairperson of the department of physical medicine and rehabilitation at the Millcreek Community Hospital and the Veterans Affairs Medical Center in Erie, Pennsylvania, and is also chief of rehabilitation services at Great Lakes Rehabilitation Hospital in Erie.

Since 1992, Dr. Ferretti has been the provost, senior vice president, and dean of academic affairs of the Lake Erie College of Osteopathic Medicine. Dr. Ferretti has been on the Council of Deans of the American Association of Colleges of Osteopathic Medicine since 1993 and was the chairperson of the board of deans in 2005 and 2006. She has served as member, trustee, and officer of numerous local, state, and national organizations and institutions.

Dr. Ferretti has been the principal investigator for the Pennsylvania Generalist Physician Initiative Grant to increase the supply and distribution of primary care physicians in Pennsylvania; the American College of Family Physicians Task Force Grant 3+3 Compacted Program in Family Practice; and a Health Resources and Services Administration Grant to provide necessary and appropriate didactic and clinical training experiences to both predoctoral and graduate osteopathic family physicians.[25]

Melicien Tettambel, DO

Melicien Tettambel received her DO degree from the Kirksville College of Osteopathic Medicine in 1978. She served a rotating internship at South Bend Osteopathic Hospital and her residency in obstetrics and gynecology at Normandy Osteopathic Hospital in St. Louis, Missouri. She is board certified in obstetrics and gynecology, as well as in osteopathic manipulative medicine.

Dr. Tettambel was in the private practice of obstetrics and gynecology and osteopathic manipulative medicine for many years. She served as the chairperson of the Certifying Board of the American Osteopathic Board of Neuromusculoskeletal Medicine. She has published extensively and lectured in osteopathic colleges throughout the United States and around the world, including Russia, Australia, New Zealand, Great Britain, Canada, France, and Belgium.

She was president of the American Academy of Osteopathy and the Illinois Association of Osteopathic Physicians and Surgeons. Dr. Tettambel has also served as president of the National Osteopathic Physicians Association and was the founding president of the Illinois Osteopathic Education Foundation.

In 2004, Dr. Tettambel received the Andrew Taylor Still Medallion of Honor from the American Academy of Osteopathy. In 2006, she became president of the Sutherland Cranial Teaching Foundation. She is chairperson of Women's and

Child Health at A. T. Still University, Kirksville College of Osteopathic Medicine and practices at Northeast Regional Medical Center in Kirksville, Missouri.[26]

Carol Lynn Monson, DO

Carol Monson received her master's degree in community mental health and taught at the University of Michigan and Central Michigan University before enrolling at the Michigan State University, College of Osteopathic Medicine. She received her DO degree in 1979 and is board certified in family practice.

Dr. Monson's career has focused on making meaningful contributions to the field of medicine through teaching, education, and clinical practice in the field of osteopathic medicine. She has published extensively and in 1997 received the writing award for the Outstanding Scientific Paper by the American College of Osteopathic Family Physicians. She is an accomplished and sought-after lecturer on multiple subjects in the field of family practice.

Dr. Monson is a professor of family medicine at Michigan State University, College of Osteopathic Medicine. She is active in the intern and residency training programs at the university and serves as medical director for the Family and Community Medicine Clinic. She maintains active hospital privileges in the Department of Family Medicine at the Ingham Regional Medical Center and Sparrow Hospital in Lansing, Michigan.[27]

Karen J. Nichols, DO

Karen J. Nichols started her career as a medical technologist. She obtained her master's degree in health care administration, and then in 1981 received her DO degree from the University of Health Sciences, College of Osteopathic Medicine, Kansas City. She served her internship and residency in internal medicine at the Oklahoma Osteopathic Hospital, where she was chief resident.

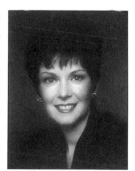

Karen J. Nichols, DO

Dr. Nichols had a private internal medicine and geriatrics practice in Mesa, Arizona, from 1985 until 2002. She served a Health Policy Fellowship from 1995 to 1996. She received an honorary doctorate of humane letters from University of Health Sciences, College of Osteopathic Medicine, Kansas City in 2001 and was a Costin Scholar at Chicago College of Osteopathic Medicine from 2004 to 2005. Dr. Nichols has held numerous academic positions, and in 2002 she became dean of the Chicago College of Osteopathic Medicine of Midwestern University.

Dr. Nichols has received numerous awards, including the first Arizona Osteopathic Medical Association Physician of the Year Award. She has served as president of the Arizona Osteopathic Association and president of the American College of Osteopathic Internists. Dr. Nichols has served on the boards of the Kansas City University of Medicine and Biosciences College of Osteopathic Medicine and the American Osteopathic Foundation.[28]

Dr. Nichols is a member of the Board of Trustees of the American Osteopathic Association. She is the founding chairperson of the AOA End of Life Care Advisory Committee and serves on multiple other committees. On 18 July 2009, Dr. Nichols was elected president of the AOA, the first woman elected to this high position.[29]

Sister Anne Brooks, SNJM, DO

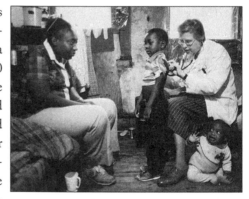

Sister Anne Brooks, SNJM, DO [photo by Andy Levin, 1987]

In the 1980s, Tutwiler was, and remains today, a depressed town of 1,200 people in the Mississippi Delta with a per capita income of less than $3,000 a year, an infant mortality rate more than twice the national average, and rampant illiteracy, malnutrition, and disease. Most homes lacked indoor plumbing, and raw sewage contaminated the bayou that ran through the town. When the Harvard University Physician Task Force on Hunger in America visited Tutwiler, they reported, "We really saw people as close to survival as one is likely to find in this nation." Although the town council had run repeated ads in medical journals trying to attract a physician, the town had not had a physician for many years. Then in 1983, the mayor received a letter from a physician who wanted to establish a medical practice in Tutwiler. That physician was Sister Anne Brooks, DO. When the stunned mayor asked why a Catholic nun would want to come to a town that had no Catholics she replied, "I was looking for the bottom of the barrel and Tutwiler is it."

Since 1983, Sister Anne Brooks, along with four other nuns (each from a different order) who work with her in the Tutwiler Clinic have dedicated their lives to serving the poor and medically underserved patients of Mississippi. The clinic charges only what the patient can afford to pay and 70 percent of the patients cannot afford to pay anything, so the clinic survives mostly on donations from caring people throughout the country. Sister Anne Brooks is the medical director and for many years was the only physician. In 2007, a second physician joined the clinic to help with the large numbers of patients. Sister Maureen runs the community education center a block away from the clinic, Sister Joanne is the clinic counselor, and Sister Cora Lee is the clinic coordinator, managing the thirty employees and annual patient load of 8,500. The clinic also provides part-time dental, optometry, and podiatry services. Sister Eileen is a nurse practitioner who operated a satellite clinic fifteen miles from the primary clinic until it was forced to close in October 2010 due to lack of funding, after sixteen years of service to the community. To this day, the sisters remain the only Catholics in Tutweiler and must travel to the next county to attend church services.

Sr. Anne Brooks joined the Sisters of the Holy Names of Jesus and Mary (SNJM) in 1955 in Rome, New York, attending the St. Bonaventure University Extension at the Novitiate. From 1957 until 1973, Sr. Anne taught elementary school and was director of the St. Petersburg (Florida) Free Clinic from 1973 to 1977. Sr. Anne was diagnosed with severe rheumatoid arthritis and had been confined to a wheelchair for several years when John Upledger, DO, began treating her. As Sr. Anne's health improved, Dr. Upledger challenged her to pursue a career in osteopathic medicine, leading to her acceptance at Michigan State University, College of Osteopathic Medicine at age forty. Sr. Anne graduated in 1982 and served a rotating internship at the Riverside Osteopathic Hospital in Trenton, Michigan. Over the years, Sr. Anne has been given awards and recognition by multiple groups and organizations for her selfless dedication to providing medical care to the poor of Mississippi. Donations generated from public response to the awards have enabled the clinic to stay open, with charitable contributions accounting for 75 percent of the funds needed to keep the clinic running. To the religious community she is Sr. Anne and in the medical community she is called Dr. Brooks, but to her clinic patients, she is affectionately called Daboo.

Dr. Sr. Anne Brooks is the first to recognize the contributions of the other nuns and staff of the clinic for their combined efforts to "empower our own patients to take charge of their health and lives," thus continuing the challenge and inspiration that formed the basis of her own ability to follow her osteopathic calling.[30]

Diane Marilyn Bourlier, DO

Practicing pediatric emergency medicine in a large urban pediatric trauma center is just what Dr. Diane Bourlier does every working day. A graduate of the Kansas City College of Osteopathic Medicine of the University of Health Sciences in 1987, Dr. Bourlier served her internship at the Oklahoma Osteopathic Hospital, her pediatric residency at the Arnold Palmer Hospital for Children and Women, and her pediatric emergency medicine fellowship at the Miami Children's Hospital.

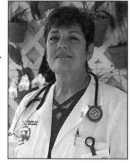

Diane M. Bourlier, DO

Prior to going back to college and medical school, Dr. Bourlier was an RN and worked as an operating room charge nurse. She has bachelor degrees in English and philosophy and has published articles including "Pediatric Office Emergencies," "Snakebites," and "Trauma to Children from Riding atop Moving Vehicles." When not providing pediatric emergency care, she spends her time teaching pediatric acute life support and lecturing on emergency care to resident physicians. She has been actively involved in pediatric trauma and child abuse programs. Dr. Bourlier is presently a pediatric emergency physician at St. Joseph's Hospital, Children's Emergency Department in Tampa, Florida.[31]

Jill B. Vosler, DO

Jill Vosler, DO, is a board-certified family practitioner residing in Eaton, Ohio, where she has lived for the majority of her life, leaving only to acquire her undergraduate and graduate education. She obtained a bachelor's degree in psychology from Miami University and then went to Ohio University College of Osteopathic Medicine, where she obtained her DO in 1988. Dr. Vosler has been in practice for many years in the same building with two of her brothers. Her father retired from family practice, and she has a brother practicing family medicine in Arizona.

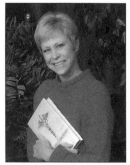

Jill B. Vosler, DO

Along with maintaining a busy family practice, Dr. Vosler serves as the Eaton High School team physician, is on the Preble County Mental Health and Recovery Board, and is the president of the Eaton Little League. She has recently pursued a path as an author and published her first book, *Legal Larceny*, where she explores what would happen if doctors across the

United States, tired of endless litigation and skyrocketing malpractice costs, simply decided to quit. She hopes to write several more books in the near future.[32]

Jane Elizabeth Carreiro, DO

Jane Elizabeth Carreiro, DO, graduated from the University of New England College of Osteopathic Medicine in 1988. She completed her internship at Waterville Osteopathic Hospital, served a pediatric residency at Nassau County Medical Center, and served a family practice residency at the Waterville Osteopathic Hospital.

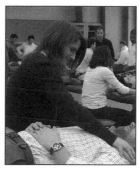

Jane Elizabeth Carreiro, DO

Dr. Jane Carreiro is associate professor and chair of the Department of Osteopathic Manipulative Medicine at New England College of Osteopathic Medicine in Biddleford, Maine. She is board certified in family practice and osteopathic manipulative medicine. In addition to medicine, her academic pursuits include human dissection, functional anatomy, and clinical neurophysiology. Dr. Carreiro's clinical practice is primarily osteopathic pediatrics.

Dr. Carreiro lectures throughout the United States, Europe, and Australia. She holds visiting faculty positions at the Wiener Schule für Osteopathie, the Deutsche Gesellschaft für Osteopathische Medizin, the Deutsche American Osteopathische Association, and the Royal Melbourne Technology University. She serves on the faculty of the Sutherland Cranial Teaching Foundation and is a member of the Still-Sutherland Study Group. Dr. Carreiro serves as vice president on the executive board of the World Osteopathic Health Organization. She holds leadership positions in the American Academy of Osteopathy and has authored the *International Guidelines for Osteopathic Training and Practice* for the World Health Organization. Dr. Carreiro is the author of *An Osteopathic Approach to Children,* which has been translated into French, German, and Italian.[33]

Debra A. Smith, DO

Dr. Debra A. Smith is chief medical officer for International Medical Group/Akeso Care Management, which provides international medical insurance and medical evacuation. Among her multiple responsibilities, she has reengineered the medical evacuation process for her company's travel and expatriate customers around the world; she is directly involved in coordinating evacuations.

Dr. Smith received her doctorate in osteopathic medicine from the Nova Southeastern University, College of Osteopathic Medicine in Ft. Lauderdale, Florida, in 1993. She also holds masters degrees in business administration and in international health management from the Thunderbird School of Global Management. She served her residency in public health and general preventive medicine at the Emory University School of Medicine in Atlanta, Georgia. She trained at the Centers for Disease Control and Preven-

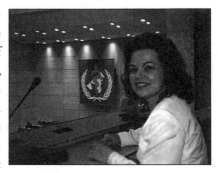

Debra A. Smith, DO, MIHM, MBA, at the World Health Assembly, Geneva, Switzerland

tion and holds a certificate in tropical medicine and public health from the Johns Hopkins University, School of Hygiene and Public Health.

Dr. Smith is board certified in public health and general preventive medicine by both the American Board of Preventive Medicine and the American Osteopathic Board of Preventive Medicine. She has served as a health financing consultant for the World Bank in the former Soviet republic of Georgia and a public health consultant for the United Nations High Commissioner for Refugees in the former Soviet republic of South Ossetia.

Dr. Smith was the first to propose the formation of the Osteopathic International Alliance in speeches at the 1999 and 2000 national conventions of the American Osteopathic Association. From 2003 to 2006 she served on the founding board of directors of the Osteopathic International Alliance. From 2004 to 2006, Dr. Smith was chairman of the American Osteopathic Association's Strategic Planning Committee, Bureau of International Osteopathic Medical Education and Affairs. On multiple occasions she has served as a delegate for the American Osteopathic Association and the Global Health Council to the World Health Organization's annual assembly in Geneva, Switzerland. Responding to "politicians attempting to hijack healthcare for their own gain," in 2009 Dr. Smith published *Healthcare Solved: Real Answers, No Politics*.[34]

Sonia Rivera-Martinez, DO

Sonia Rivera-Martinez was born in an impoverished neighborhood in the Bronx, New York. When she was a child, her father's illness took the family back to Puerto Rico where her mother's family lived. In 1983, she graduated magna cum laude from the University of Puerto Rico with a degree in accounting and finance. While in college, she received many honors, including induction into the University of Puerto Rico Honor Society and the Business Administration Honor Society.

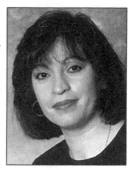

Sonia Rivera-Martinez, DO

Rivera-Martinez returned to New York and established a successful career as a controller. Years later, while volunteering at a local hospital, she made the decision to change careers. In 1997, after she had already become a grandmother, with the support of her husband and family, she enrolled at the New York College of Osteopathic Medicine. While a student, Rivera-Martinez was awarded the Osteopathic Manipulative Medicine Predoctoral Fellowship. In 2001 she cofounded the Project for Latino Health, New York College of Osteopathic Medicine Chapter of the National Boricua Latino Health Organization. She also worked as a research and teaching assistant, was treasurer of her medical school class, and served, at various times, as president, vice president, and secretary of the school's chapter of the National Undergraduate Fellows Association.

Since graduating in 2002, Dr. Rivera-Martinez was named Long Beach Medical Center Intern of the Year. She has also been awarded the National Health Service Corps Scholarship Graduate Award and the New York Institute of Technology Presidential Service Award two times, among other awards.

In her short career as a physician, Dr. Rivera-Martinez has been prolific in medical research. She has published four papers and five abstracts in the *Journal of the American Osteopathic Association* and the *American Academy of Osteopathy Journal*, and has made fourteen presentations on the national level. Her work has included studies on the forces used during osteopathic manipulation, cranial dysfunctions in patients with Parkinson's disease, and the biomechanics of the cervical spine. She is a contributing author of *An Osteopathic Approach to Diagnosis and Treatment*, 3rd ed., and also edited *The Collected Writings of Robert G. Thorpe, DO, FAAO*. Dr. Rivera-Martinez is the principal investigator of two studies on the interexaminer reliability of diagnostic palpation, and is coinvestigator of a study on the osteopathic treatment of hypothyroid patients; additional studies are in the initial stages.

When she started on her new career in medicine, Rivera-Martinez promised herself that she would return to her roots and assist those who have difficulty obtaining adequate medical care. Making good on this promise, she has made a four-year commitment to the National Health Service Corps to provide services to the medically underserved population.

At the urging of Dr. Rivera-Martinez, the American Osteopathic Association sent a petition to the Board of Medical Examiners in Puerto Rico for recognition of the Comprehensive Osteopathic Medical Licensing Examination so that American-trained osteopathic physicians could obtain full unrestricted licenses in Puerto Rico. After a year went by without a reply, Dr. Rivera-Martinez appeared before the Board of Medical Examiners of Puerto Rico to inquire if the board required additional information and to present arguments in favor of the petition. As of spring 2011, the board's decision is still pending and Dr. Rivera-Martinez is lobbying for support from the Puerto Rico Medical Association.

Dr. Rivera-Martinez's accomplishments in such a short time are greater than the lifetime accomplishments of many physicians, and are even more remarkable in light of the fact that, as of spring 2011, she is only in the second year of her family practice residency at the Long Beach Medical Center in Long Beach, New York, where she is the assistant chief resident of the Department of Family Medicine.[35]

Rosanna Sabini, DO

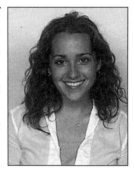

Rosanna Sabini, DO

While a medical student at the New York College of Osteopathic Medicine, Rosanna Sabini was chief predoctoral teaching fellow in osteopathic manipulative medicine. After receiving her DO degree in 2005, Sabini served a traditional osteopathic rotating internship at Long Beach Medical Center and went on to her residency in physical medicine and rehabilitation at Mount Sinai Medical Center.

Dr. Sabini's list of publications in peer-reviewed journals is already significant, including articles and abstracts in the *Journal of the American Osteopathic Association*, *Rehab Review*, and *Biological Chemistry*. Research is yet another part of Dr. Sabini's professional accomplishments. She has participated in many and varied research projects, including studies on the use of Botox, the effects of Rosiglitazone (diabetic medication) on cellular proteins, and the morphology and clinical significance of cranial sutures. As of spring 2011, she is researching "Coupled Motions of the Spine" with Sonia Rivera-Martinez, DO, and the "Tactile Sensation of Osteopaths" with Charles Smutny, DO.

A fluent speaker of Italian, Dr. Sabini has lectured on various subjects, including osteopathy in Italy, and has been an active volunteer in her community.[36]

Andrea Jones, DO

Graduation from medical school is a memorable occasion for anyone, but for Andrea Jones, a 2006 graduate from the Kirksville College of Osteopathic Medicine, graduation was truly remarkable. Andrea had looked forward to the day she would walk across the stage to receive her DO diploma, but that was not to happen for her. At the awards banquet the evening before graduation, Andrea went into labor, two weeks early. With her husband at her side, she delivered a healthy baby girl, Lilly Sophia Jones, and was in the hospital at the time she should have been receiving her long-awaited and hard-earned diploma. Much to Andrea's surprise, Dean Slocum, Dean Laird, Dean Subedits, and Professor Smith brought graduation to the hospital instead. Dr. Jones's reaction was, "She [Lily] is the best graduation gift I could have received."[37]

Robyn Kratenstein

While in high school, Robyn Kratenstein played field hockey for four years, was on the swimming and diving team for three years, and was on the track team for one year. While a student at Salisbury University in Maryland, she played on the girls' ultimate Frisbee team for four years and was team captain for one year. This sounds like a typical athletic college student, until one realizes that Robyn was born without her left hand and the lower portion of her left arm. When playing field hockey, she wore a special device she and her coach had designed so she could hold the hockey stick. Robyn says, "If anyone

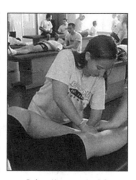

Robyn Kratenstein, DO

were to meet me and get to know me they would of course notice that I have only one hand. But after spending more time with me they would realize that although my experiences due to my arm have shaped me, it is not my arm that defines me. I am driven by the desire to help people and my love and curiosity for medicine. Most of my friends no longer notice that I have only one hand, but they do notice that I am a driven, fun-loving, honest, and caring person!"

While in college, Kratenstein became a member of Kappa Delta Pi (educational honor society) and Beta Beta Beta (biological honor society). She graduated from Salisbury University cum laude with a degree in biology and elementary education.

She studied education not because she wanted to be a teacher but because she felt the degree would be of assistance in her planned career as a pediatrician.

Robyn has known since she was in high school that she wanted to become a physician and when it came time to apply to medical school, Robyn applied only to osteopathic medical colleges, "because I believe in the osteopathic philosophy of treating the whole person." After receiving her DO degree from Lake Erie College of Osteopathic Medicine, Bradenton in 2010, she began her residency as an emergency room physician at Conemangh Memorial Hospital in Johnstown, Pennsylvania.[38]

Christy L. Nolan, DO

Starting with Andrew Taylor Still's own family, osteopathic medicine has had many "osteopathic families" and this tradition continues to this day. Christy Nolan is the newest member of one of those traditionally osteopathic families. When she entered the Lake Erie College of Osteopathic Medicine–Bradenton as a member of the class of 2010, Christy became the fourth generation of her family to enter osteopathic medicine.

Christy's great-grandfather Fredrick C. Wirt started the tradition as a 1910 graduate of the American School of Osteopathy. Her great-grandmother Hazel's cousin K. C. Davis, DO, was dean of the osteopathic college in Kansas City, Missouri. While Fred was still a student, he and Hazel had their first child, delivered at the osteopathic hospital by Dr. Andrew T. Still. After receiving his DO degree, Fred Wirt moved to Florida and became the first DO to establish a practice in Pasco County.

Dr. Fredrick and Hazel Wirt had four children. Their second daughter, Margaret (Peg) Wirt, became a DO general practitioner and married John (Jack) Tedrick, DO, a radiologist. They were both graduates of the Kansas City College of Osteopathy and Surgery. Their third child, Wenton (Sandy) Wirt, DO, graduated from Kansas City College of Osteopathy and Surgery and practiced general medicine in Crystal River, Florida. Their youngest son, Philip Richard Wirt, did not become a DO, but his two sons both became osteopathic physicians.

Philip Wirt's older son, Philip Richard Wirt III graduated from Kansas City College of Osteopathic Medicine in 1978 and is board certified in family practice. As he was preparing to follow the family tradition, his grandmother, Hazel, advised him: "No matter what special interest you follow in your medical career, make sure that you become a Ten-Fingered Osteopath." His second son, Robert C. Wirt, graduated from Kansas City College of Osteopathic Medicine in 1983, is board certified in family practice, and practices in Gainesville, Georgia.

Philip Wirt III's daughter, Christy Nolan, graduated from Lake Erie College of Osteopathic Medicine, Bradenton in 2010, exactly one hundred years after her great-grandfather graduated from the American School of Osteopathy.[39]

Elena Choumkina Vrotsos, DO

In 2001, Elena Choumkina arrived in the United States from Kazakhstan. She had studied in Russian schools in Chelyabinsk and Dubna, a region close to Moscow, but her childhood dream of becoming a physician could not be fulfilled under Russian rule. When she arrived in the United States, Elena was twenty years old and had the equivalent of a high-school education; she had only US$500, knew no one, and could not speak English.

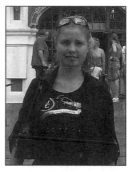

Elena Choumkina Vrotsos, DO

In her first year in her adopted country, she worked as a housekeeper, a dishwasher, and a kitchen helper, managing to save enough money to enroll at Valencia Community College. At her first opportunity, she transferred to the University of Central Florida. In the summer of 2004, she earned a scholarship and obtained a position in a research laboratory. While still attending college, she presented the results of her research on a new drug for the treatment of Alzheimer's disease at the University of Central Florida Showcase of Undergraduate Research Excellence and presented a second paper at the Society of Neuroscience in Washington, DC.

In 2005, while working full time in the research laboratory, learning to speak a new language, and struggling to learn the customs of her new country, Elena graduated from University of Central Florida with honors in molecular biology. In August 2006, she started medical school at the Lake Erie College of Osteopathic Medicine, Bradenton in Florida and received her DO degree in 2010. As of spring 2011, Elena is a pathology resident at Mount Sinai Medical Center in Miami Beach, Florida.[40]

Miranda Tsukamoto McGahan, Class of 2014

Miranda Tsukamoto and Mike McGahan began dating in their freshman year at Olympia High School in Orlando, Florida. They spoke frequently about their plans for the future, sharing their life's ambitions. Miranda had visions of serving her fellow man by becoming an osteopathic physician and Mike planned to serve his country as a military officer, and they strongly supported each other's dreams.

Mike graduated from the University of Florida in August 2008 and enrolled in the Army Officers Candidate School at Fort Benning, Georgia. In April 2009, he was commissioned a second lieutenant, and after completing advanced training as a combat engineer, was assigned as a platoon leader in the 101st Airborne Division. In August 2009, Mike and Miranda became engaged and were married on 27 November 2009, just weeks before Miranda graduated from the University of Florida.

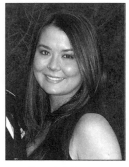

Miranda Tsukamoto
McGahan

The newlyweds celebrated Miranda's acceptance to medical school just weeks before Mike's deployment to Afghanistan, but as Miranda was preparing for life as a medical student, she received the devastating news that Mike had been killed in an ambush on 6 June 2010. Second Lieutenant Michael McGahan was awarded the Bronze Star and the Purple Heart for his service to his country, and was buried with honors at Arlington National Cemetery on 28 June 2010.

After much internal turmoil, Miranda decided that Mike, who had always supported her plans for medical school, would have wanted her to continue, and so in July 2010, Miranda McGahan became a member of the class of 2014 at the Lake Erie College of Osteopathic Medicine–Bradenton, following the dream she had so frequently shared with Mike.[41]

NOTES

1. *AOA Fact Sheet*, 1965; and *AOA Fact Sheet*, 2006.

2. Baker, "Female Enrollment in Colleges of Osteopathic Medicine," *JAOA* 95, no. 10 (Oct. 1991): 604–6.

3. Gevitz, *The DOs*, 147–48.

4. Berge et al., "Osteopathy: Special Report of the Judicial Council to the AMA House of Delegates," *JAMA* 177, no. 11 (1961): 774–76.

5. Gevitz, *The DOs*, 143–44.

6. "Michigan to Establish Osteopathic School," *AOA News Review* 12 (Aug. 1969): 1–2.

7. Gevitz, *The DOs*, 152.

8. "TCOM Becomes State-Supported Medical School," *Texas Osteopathic Physicians Journal* 32 (July 1975): 12–13.

9. AOA, "Medical Licensure Statistics for 1970," *JAMA* 216, no. 11 (14 June 1971): 1786.

10. AOA, "Years States Passed Unlimited Practice Laws"; and Wright, *Perspectives in Osteopathic Medicine*, 5.

11. See Osborne, *History of the Oklahoma State University College of Osteopathic Medicine*; and Thiessen, "Greenbriar: The Little College that Could."

12. "California Reopens to DOs," *The DO* 14 (May 1974): 81.

13. American Association of Colleges of Osteopathic Medicine, *2006 Annual Statistical Report on Osteopathic Medical Education*, table 5.

14. Licciardone and Herron, "Characteristics, Satisfaction, and Perceptions of Patients Receiving Ambulatory Healthcare from Osteopathic Physicians," *JAOA* 101 (July 2001): 374–85.

15. *AOA Fact Sheet*, 2006.

16. Urban and Rural Systems Associates, *Women in Osteopathic Medicine*, table 3, pp. 17–22.

17. Simpson and Weiser, "Studying the Impact of Women on Osteopathic Physician Workforce Predictions," *JAOA* 96, no. 2 (Feb. 1996): 109–10.

18. Potee, Gerber, and Ickovics, "Medicine and Motherhood: Shifting Trends among Female Physicians from 1922 to 1999," *Academic Medicine* 74, no. 8 (Aug. 1999): 911–14.

19. Sexton, "Working 9 to 3," *Florida Medical Business* 22, no. 9 (May 2008): 1–12.

20. DiGiovanna, *Encyclopedia of Osteopathy*, 35.

21. Pauline Schultz, DO, personal correspondence with the author, 13 November 2006.

22. "ACOS Inaugurates New President during Annual Ceremonial Conclave," *ACOS News* 44, no. 12 (Oct. 2006): 1–5.

23. Barbara Ross-Lee, DO, personal correspondence with the author, 31 October 2006.

24. Virginia Syperda, DO, personal correspondence with the author, 31 October 2006 and 7 August 2009.

25. Silvia Ferretti, DO, personal correspondence with the author, 4 May 2007.

26. Melicien Tettambel, DO, personal correspondence with the author, 2 December 2006.

27. Carol Monson, DO, personal correspondence with the author, 7 December 2006.

28. Karen Nichols, DO, personal correspondence with the author, 18 December 2006.

29. *AOA Daily Report,* 19 July 2009.

30. Sr. Anne Brooks, DO, personal correspondence with the author, 4 February 2011.

31. Diane Bourlier, DO, personal correspondence with the author, 25 March 2007.

32. Jill Vosler, DO, personal correspondence with the author, 24 February 2007.

33. Jane Carreiro, DO, personal correspondence with the author, 27 November 2006.

34. Debra Smith, personal correspondence with the author, 24 April 2008.

35. Sonia Rivera-Martinez, personal correspondence with the author, 26 January 2007.

36. Rosanna Sabini, DO, personal correspondence with the author, 5 February 2007.

37. "New Arrival Makes for Unique Graduation, KCOM Graduate Delivers Baby on Commencement Day," *Still News* (July 2005): 5.

38. Robyn Kratenstein, personal correspondence with the author, 23 March 2007.

39. Christy Nolan, personal correspondence with the author, 17 June 2007; and information from Philip Richard Wirt III, DO.

40. Elena Choumkina Vrotsos, DO, personal correspondence with the author, 30 November 2007.

41. Miranda Tsukamoto McGahan, personal correspondence with the author, 5 January 2011.

Chapter Six

Women in Osteopathic Research

"Dr. Still respected the fact that women possess a fine palpatory touch."

Mary McClellan Burnett, DO

"In the unfolding of the new system of healing, osteopathy, there has been offered to women, such an opportunity as never before in any profession, because of her temperament, by the general fineness of texture of her makeup, she is particularly apt in acquiring the *discriminating touch* and the deftness of movement so necessary in the osteopathic operator."

Ellen Barret Ligon, DO

FROM THE VERY BEGINNING, research has played a fundamental role in the osteopathic profession. Dr. A. T. Still developed his theories of osteopathic medicine through his study of the anatomy and physiology of the human body. His years of methodical research led him to an understanding of the interaction of form and structure and its effect on the human body, of the body's inherent ability to regulate and heal itself, and of the importance of treating the person as a whole being.[1]

Even after Dr. Still opened the American School of Osteopathy (ASO), he continued to study and expand on his techniques. Early publications of the school mention research projects as early as 1896, but documentation of this research no longer exists.[2] Dr. William Smith, who had teamed with Dr. Still to open the ASO, was the first physician in America to inject contrast material into the arterial system to outline the blood vessels, conducting his research at the ASO. He named his procedure skiagraphy, but today this procedure is known as angiography. He published "Skiagraphy and the Circulation" in the *American X-Ray Journal* in December 1898.[3] Also in 1898, Drs. John Littlejohn and C. Hulett performed experiments on the effects of manipulative therapy in relationship to spinal manipulation.[4]

Between 1904 and 1914, osteopathic research was conducted at the Pacific College of Osteopathy under the capable leadership of Louisa Burns, DO. Prior to 1913, all osteopathic research was performed by the osteopathic medical schools and by individual DOs. In 1911 the American Osteopathic Association (AOA) took action to promote and finance a profession-wide coordinated research program, and in 1913, the A. T. Still Research Institute opened in Chicago, with John Deason, DO, serving as director. The Still Research Institute provided the osteopathic profession with a place to conduct basic research and to teach advanced courses on osteopathic manipulative medicine to practicing DOs. The institute's second and most famous director was Louisa Burns, DO, the profession's first full-time researcher. Dr. Burns dedicated her long and productive research career to the study of the effects of manipulative therapy on different systems of the human body.[5]

In 1917, a California branch of the research institute was established, and the new Sunny Slope Laboratory became the center for osteopathic research under the direction of Dr. Burns when the original laboratory in Chicago was closed in 1918. In 1925, the facility was expanded to accommodate the growing research programs.[6] In 1950, the facility was renamed the Louisa Burns Osteopathic Research Laboratory and moved to the campus of the College of Osteopathic Physicians and Surgeons in Los Angeles.

In addition to the research facility supported primarily by the AOA and individual DOs, each osteopathic medical college continued to fund research at its own institution. There was no outside funding for this early osteopathic research. It was not until 1947 that an osteopathic institution first received a federal research grant. In that year, the Kirksville College of Osteopathy and Surgery received a grant for $6,119 from the US Public Health Service for research to be conducted by J. S. Denslow, DO.[7]

In 1961, the Louisa Burns Osteopathic Research Laboratory was lost to the profession when the College of Osteopathic Physicians and Surgeons converted to an allopathic medical college. This was a crippling blow to osteopathic research, from which the profession would not completely recover until 2001, when the Osteopathic Research Center, an autonomous unit within the University of North Texas Health Science Center, was established with the mission of conducting nationwide collaborative research on the efficacy of osteopathic manipulative medicine. In addition to funding from osteopathic associations, the Osteopathic Research Center has received funding from the National Institute of Health and conducts multicenter research projects.[8]

INFLUENZA PANDEMIC OF 1918/19

The influenza pandemic of 1918/19 provided a unique opportunity for osteopathic physicians to study the effectiveness of their treatments. The pandemic killed an estimated 500,000 to 650,000 people in the United States alone.[9] During the height of the pandemic in 1919, osteopathic researchers carried out a retrospective cohort research study, which revealed that of influenza patients being treated by osteopathic physicians, only one out of four hundred died, whereas patients treated by other physicians had a death rate of twenty out of four hundred.[10] Even patients who had developed pneumonia as a secondary complication had a much greater chance of living if they were treated by a DO.

In the absence of modern medications, such as antibiotics and antiviral medications, and the advanced life support apparatus now available, osteopathic physicians used the resources available to them at the time, primarily manipulative therapy.[11] Following the flu pandemic, many theories were forwarded to explain the success of osteopathic treatments. Some stated that the osteopathic care inhibited the sympathetic nervous system, decreasing the secretion of mucus,[12] others speculated that the osteopathic treatments stimulated the adrenal gland,[13] and some speculated that it was medications administered by MDs that had been detrimental to their patients.[14]

In 2006, research carried out at the Osteopathic Research Center at the University of North Texas Health Science Center found that osteopathic manipulation dramatically increases the flow of lymphatic fluid, draining the lungs of congestion and increasing the number of disease-fighting white blood cells in the lymphatic fluid. This boosts the body's immune system, enabling the patient to survive the crisis period and allowing the body's self-healing mechanisms to function.[15]

Another type of research focused on examining the claims of inventors who advertised devices to treat the musculoskeletal system. Most of these devices were inefficient forms of traction or purported to correct posture. They were variously described as massage machines, vibrating machines, rolling machines, mechanical stimulators, pummeling machines, or muscle beaters. In fact, most had minimal or no actual benefit to the patient.[16] Investigations by both osteopathic and allopathic physicians quickly revealed the worthlessness of these machines, and in a rare instance of cooperation, MDs joined DOs in condemning these useless devices.

In the early twentieth century, there was a short-lived period of enthusiasm for the electric theories of medicine, which were based on the theories of Albert Abrams, MD, called the Electronic Reactions of Abrams (ERA).[17] Abrams, a native of San Francisco and one-time vice president of the California State Medical Society, theorized that all diseases have a vibratory rate specific to the disease and that this vibration can be measured. He claimed that his machine would diagnose disease by detecting the rate of vibration of a drop of the patient's blood. He also developed the "Oscilloclast" to treat disease with vibrations. Scientific and medical journals were filled with letters both extolling and decrying the theories of ERA, and dozens of electronic medical schools opened throughout the country to teach ERA. After J. V. McManis, DO, inventor of the McManis Table for manipulative therapy, opened an electronic medical school in Missouri, the Missouri State Osteopathic Board adopted a resolution opposing the practice of ERA until it could be proven scientifically and requested the two osteopathic colleges to investigate and do research on electronic medicine.[18]

At the request of the Missouri State Osteopathic Board, Dr. Laughlin of the Andrew Taylor Still College of Osteopathy and Surgery and Dr. Waggoner of the ASO conducted research on the use of electric medicine to determine if it was based on scientific principles. After independent investigations, in 1923 both osteopathic researchers separately concluded that there was insufficient scientific evidence to justify the use of ERA and labeled it a hoax that should not be used by osteopathic physicians.[19] The McManis School of Electronic Medicine closed shortly after the osteopathic colleges announced the results of their research. The following year, in September 1924, the magazine *Scientific American* published a study by a group of allopathic physicians and physicists that also denounced electronic medicine and the ERA theory. The AMA labeled Dr. Abrams the "dean of twentieth-century charlatans." The ERA scam is considered by many to be the greatest medical hoax of all time.[20]

During the early and middle years of the osteopathic profession, improving the quality of osteopathic medical education was the major focus of attention, while research was invariably relegated to a minor position because of the lack of funding. Starting in the mid-1980s, however, research has received increased attention throughout the profession, enhanced by the availability of government and university funding and research grants previously unavailable to the profession.[21] The AOA has made research a priority in all osteopathic institutions of higher learning. This research is not restricted to verification of the osteopathic approach, but includes all segments of medical and basic science research, including cancer, AIDS, cardiovascular disease, infectious disease, and a multiplicity of other research programs. In the last quarter century, osteopathic research on the validity of osteopathic diagnosis and treatment has focused on: 1. reliability of interexaminer agreement of diagnostic findings; 2. precise measurement of somatic dysfunction with the use of instruments; and 3. correlation of physical findings throughout the body with the somatic dysfunctions found in the spine.[22]

DO and DO/PhD researchers stand side by side with MD and PhD researchers in general medical research, but when it comes to verification of osteopathic principles, the osteopathic profession itself must define and enumerate what the profession stands for. A notable exception is the study published in the *New England Journal of Medicine* in 1999 that compared osteopathic manipulative therapy with standard medical treatment for patients with low back pain. This collaborative study by the Departments of Orthopedic Surgery and Preventive Medicine of Rush-Presbyterian-St. Luke's Medical Center and the Chicago College of Osteopathic Medicine revealed that although final outcomes demonstrated no statistical difference between the two groups and 90 percent of the patients from both groups were satisfied with the results of their care, patients receiving osteopathic manipulative therapy required significantly less medication. Patients treated by the MD orthopedic surgeons required thirteen times more physical therapy and significantly greater quantities of painkillers, anti-inflammatory agents, and muscle relaxant medications.[23]

The conclusions of this and similar studies notwithstanding, no matter how closely osteopathic manipulative therapy is identified with the osteopathic profession, it does not exclusively define the principles of osteopathic medicine, which the AOA defines as "a complete system of medical care with a philosophy that combines the needs of the patient with the current practice of medicine, surgery, and obstetrics; that emphasizes the interrelationship between structure and function; and which has an appreciation of the body's ability to heal itself."

To encourage medical research among osteopathic medical students, osteopathic universities have chapters of the Student Osteopathic Research Association and six osteopathic universities offer DO/PhD programs for students interested in pursuing research and teaching careers.[24] In addition to the AOA research conference held at the organization's annual convention, there is an annual international conference on osteopathic research. The first conference was held in 1999 in London and most of these conferences have been held in Europe.

Women in Research
Lillian Whiting, DO

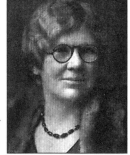

Lillian Whiting, DO
[1944 *Clinical Osteopathy*, MOM]

Lillian Whiting graduated from the Pacific College of Osteopathy in 1903. While running an active obstetrics practice in Los Angeles, Dr. Whiting conducted research that found that women who received osteopathic manipulative therapy (OMT) routinely during their first pregnancy had their labor shortened by over two-thirds compared with women who had not received OMT during their pregnancy. Those women receiving OMT had an average labor of nine hours, fifty-four minutes; those not receiving OMT had an average labor of twenty-one hours, six minutes.

Dr. Whiting also studied the length of labor for women who had previous deliveries. Her findings were similar; those who received OMT during their pregnancy had shorter labor times than those who had not received OMT. Dr. Whiting published her findings in the *Journal of the American Osteopathic Association* (vol. 11, 1912). In her article titled "Can the Length of Labor be Shortened by Osteopathic Treatment?" Dr. Whiting concluded that OMT had shortened the duration of labor.

Louisa Burns, DO

Following graduation from college, Louisa Burns became a schoolteacher, but her career was cut short when she developed spinal meningitis. Although she survived, Louisa was severely debilitated by the effects of the disease. Gaining no relief from the regular medical therapies of the time, in desperation she turned to osteopathy. Attributing her remarkable recovery to the osteopathic treatments she received, Burns was so impressed that she enrolled in an osteopathic medical school.

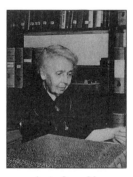

Louisa Burns, DO
[1951 *Cortex*, MOM]

Louisa Burns graduated from the Pacific College of Osteopathy in 1904. While still an osteopathic medical student, Louisa Burns was recognized by the Southern California Academy of Sciences for her research on mold biology. Following graduation, Dr. Burns was employed for ten years as a professor of physiology at the Pacific College of Osteopathy; during that time she continued her work in research and published her first book, *Basic Principles*, in 1907.

In 1913, the A. T. Still Research Institute was established in Chicago and Dr. Burns became an enthusiastic member. In 1914, she became a full-time associate of the institute, and in 1916, she became the dean of the institute, a position she held for the next twenty years. In 1917, Dr. Louisa Burns relocated to California to become director of the newly opened Sunny Slope Laboratory, a branch of the A. T. Still Research Institute.

Louisa Burns was a prolific researcher and published numerous articles, as well as many books. She formulated the hypothesis that "the abnormal condition called a bony lesion exists and it may cause disease in distant parts of the body." Dr. Burns theorized that, "a similar condition could be produced in laboratory animals either as a disturbance in bony relations or some other pathological condition. Disease should occur in distant parts of the body of the affected animals. The correction of such bony lesions should result in at least partial recovery from the disease so produced. If the above conditions can be met, study of the tissue changes during the pathogenesis and recovery should increase our understanding of the nature of bony lesions."[25] Her most complete and extensive publication was *Studies in the Osteopathic Sciences*, a four-volume work published over a span of twenty-four years. The first volume, *Basic Principles*, was published in 1907; vol. 2, *The Nerve Centers* was published in 1911; vol. 3, *The Physiology of Consciousness*, was published in 1911; and vol. 4, *Cells of the Blood*, was published in 1931.

Dr. Burns was the first osteopathic researcher to find that there was a connection between affectations of the somatic and visceral tissue, demonstrating the existence of the somatovisceral and viscerosomatic reflexes. Louisa Burns has been recognized by the osteopathic profession as being the first DO to dedicate her life to researching the principles of osteopathy. She was a true pioneer in the field of osteopathic research and the first person ever to receive the Distinguished Service Certificate from the AOA. The Louisa Burns Memorial Lecture was established by the AOA in 1969 to honor Dr. Burns's dedicated service to her profession. This lecture is presented each year at the annual AOA Research Conference.[26]

Charlotte Weaver, DO

Charlotte Winger Weaver graduated from the ASO in 1912 with a special diploma in dissection. She practiced osteopathy most of her life in Akron, Ohio, except for the period from 1929 until 1934 when she practiced osteopathy in Paris, France. After her husband died in the influenza pandemic of 1918, she began a lifelong study of the cranium and the central nervous system. Dr. Weaver's research focused on the relationship between lesions at the base of the cranium and neuropsychiatric disorders. She regarded the bones of the cranium as modified vertebrae having articular surfaces. She did countless skull dissec-

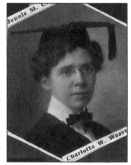

Charlotte Weaver, DO
[MOM PH 216]

tions and studies. At the time of her death at age eighty in 1964, Dr. Weaver was still working on research of the nervous system.

In 1927, the Dr. Charlotte Weaver Foundation was formed to further her original research. The foundation sponsored yearly conferences between 1927 and 1950. Her research received support from the AOA. During her long professional career, she traveled extensively doing research, studying, and practicing osteopathy.[27]

Ann E. Perry, DO

Ann E. Perry was a 1914 graduate of the Pacific College of Osteopathy.[28] She lived in Los Angeles and worked with Louisa Burns, DO, conducting research at the A. T. Still Research Institute's Clinical Research Laboratories in Los Angeles in the early twentieth century. Specializing in laboratory medicine, Dr. Perry published extensively in the *Journal of the American Osteopathic Association* and *The Western Osteopath*, focusing on the effects of OMT

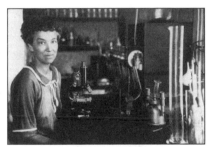

Ann E. Perry, DO, at the A. T. Still Research Institute's Clinical Research Laboratories in Los Angeles [MOM]

on laboratory findings. Dr. Perry's talents were not limited to osteopathic research and practice; she also published a collection of original poems under the title *Songs of Life*.

Beryl E. Arbuckle, DO

Beryl Arbuckle graduated from the Philadelphia College of Osteopathy in 1928. She was renowned worldwide for her research on the osteopathic cranial concept. She was a member of the Department of Pediatrics at the Philadelphia College of Osteopathy for twenty-five years.

In 1943 she worked with Dr. W. Sutherland and developed many cranial techniques for the treatment of cranial birth injuries. Dr. Arbuckle was one of the earliest researchers in the osteopathic profession to investigate and clinically test Dr. Sutherland's cranial hypotheses. She conducted

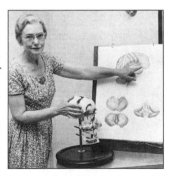

Beryl Arbuckle, DO, FAOCOP
[MOM RZ316.A73 1977]

clinical research studies in the nursery of the hospitals of the Philadelphia College of Osteopathy, in an active cranial clinic at the hospital, in her private practice, and in the anatomy laboratory where she worked with Angus G. Cathie, DO, the brilliant anatomist who developed the anatomical museum at the Philadelphia College of Osteopathic Medicine.

Dr. Arbuckle was a board-certified pediatrician and founder and director of the National Osteopathic Cerebral Palsy Foundation in Broomall, Pennsylvania. Most of her research was devoted to neurological diseases in children. Children from all over the world were brought to the Osteopathic Cerebral Palsy Foundation for evaluation and treatment.

From 1947 to 1948 she served as president of the American College of Osteopathic Pediatricians. She was awarded the Andrew Taylor Still Medallion of Honor by the American Academy of Osteopathy in 1966.

Over the years of research devoted to cranial osteopathy for children, Dr. Arbuckle has published multiple books and medical articles. In 1994, the American Academy of Osteopathy published *The Selected Writings of Beryl E. Arbuckle, DO, FAOCOP.*[29]

Miriam V. Mills, MD

Originally trained as an allopathic physician, Dr. Mills graduated from the Baylor College of Medicine in 1974. She served her internship and residency in pediatrics and a fellowship in medical geriatrics at Baylor. Although she does not have a formal degree in osteopathic medicine, Dr. Mills has over three thousand hours of continuing medical education in osteopathic manual medicine and is a clinical professor in the Department of Osteopathic Manual Medicine at the Ohio State University, College of Osteopathic Medicine. She also holds a competency certificate from the Cranial Academy.

Dr. Mills has made numerous international, national, and regional presentations on various topics in both medical and osteopathic pediatrics, and has published medical and osteopathic articles in peer-reviewed medical journals. Her original osteopathic research focused on the use of OMT to treat otitis media in children. She has received research grants from such prestigious organizations as the Robuck Fund, the Louisa Burns Osteopathic Research Committee, the Oklahoma Juvenile Authority, the AOA, and the Tulsa City County Health Department.

Commenting on her unique combination of allopathic medical training and research in osteopathic techniques, Dr. Mills asks, "Wasn't A. T. Still an MD too?"[30]

Karen M. Steele, DO

After graduating summa cum laude from Northeast Missouri State University (now Truman State University), Karen Steele received her DO degree from the Kirksville College of Osteopathic Medicine in 1974. She served a rotating internship at Eastmoreland General Hospital in Portland, Oregon, and completed a residency in osteopathic manipulative medicine at Kirksville College of Osteopathic Medicine. She is board certified in family medicine by the American Osteopathic Board of Family Practice and in osteopathic manipulative medicine by the American Osteopathic Board of Neuromuscular Medicine. She also holds a certificate of competency from the Cranial Academy.

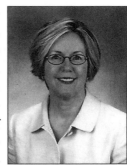

Karen Steele, DO, FAAO

Dr. Steele is a professor and associate dean for osteopathic medical education at the West Virginia School of Osteopathic Medicine. Prior to becoming an associate dean, she served as chairperson of the Division of Osteopathic Principles and Practice.

Dr. Steele has been very active in osteopathic research. She is the principal investigator of a multicenter osteopathic otitis media study, which is funded by a collaborative funding package by the National Osteopathic Research Center with grant money received from the AOA and the American Academy of Osteopathy. She has also been the principal investigator in numerous studies, including:

- Development of a research plan to investigate the efficiency of osteopathic manipulative medicine in the treatment of children with otitis media
- Effects of osteopathic manipulative medicine on gait disturbance in multiple sclerosis patients
- Effects of OMT on childhood otitis media outcomes
- Effects of OMT and neuromuscular development techniques on immobility and respiratory diseases in severely brain-damaged children
- Efficiency of OMT in the prevention of pneumonia in severely handicapped children[31]

Dr. Steele has two daughters who are also osteopathic physicians. Sarah Steele-Killian, DO, has a private practice in Salem, Virginia, and Linda Steele Roberts, DO, is a pediatric resident at the Medical College of Virginia.

Terrie Ellen Taylor, DO

Southeast Africa may not be the place one would expect to find an osteopathic physician, but osteopathic medicine is having a positive impact in Blantyre in the Republic of Malawi.

After graduating with distinction from Swarthmore College with a major in biology, Terrie Ellen Taylor received her DO degree from the Chicago College of Osteopathic Medicine in 1981, where she was class salutatorian. After an internship at the Riverside Osteopathic Hospital in Trenton, Michigan, she served her residency in internal medicine at the Detroit Osteopathic Hospital and became a fellow of the American College of Osteopathic Internists. Dr. Taylor received her master's in tropical medicine at the Liverpool School of Tropical Medicine in the United Kingdom, where she won the Glyn Williams Prize in Tropical Medicine.

From 1984 through 2000, Dr. Taylor served as codirector and, as of 2000, as director of the Blantyre Malaria Research Project at Queen Elizabeth Central Hospital in Malawi. In 2010, Dr. Taylor obtained an MRI scanner for Queen Elizabeth Central Hospital in Malawi through a grant from General Electric Corporation and the Gates Foundation. The MRI scanner was the first in Malawi and only the second in Africa.

Dr. Taylor was presented with the Young Investigator Award by the American Society of Tropical Medicine in 1987; she also received the 1996 International Health Award and the 1998 Ralph Smucker Award from Michigan State University. She was named Researcher of the Year by the American College of Osteopathic Internists in 1998 and received the Gutensohn-Denslow Award from the American Osteopathic Association Bureau of Research in 2000.

The American Society of Tropical Medicine and Hygiene awarded Dr. Taylor the Bailey K. Ashford Medal in 2006. She was named University Distinguished Professor by Michigan State University in 2006, where she is professor of tropical medicine in the College of Osteopathic Medicine.

Dr. Taylor has received many research grants over the years and is presently conducting research on severe malaria in African children for the National Institute of Allergy and Infectious Diseases. She is also researching clinicopathological correlates of cerebral malaria for the National Institute of Allergy and Infectious Diseases.[32]

In 2011, Dr. Taylor was awarded the Dr. Nathan Davis International Award in Medicine by the American Medical Association.

Sandra K. Willsie, DO

As principal investigator on thirty-five funded research projects and coinvestigator on many other research projects ranging from the treatment of diabetes to nosocomial pneumonia, it would appear that research is one of Dr. Willsie's strongest attributes. She has authored eighty-nine medical articles and abstracts. Her regional, national, and international presentations are numerous and diverse.

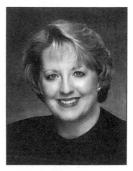

Sandra K. Willsie, DO, FACOI, FACP, FCCP

Dr. Willsie graduated from the Kansas City University of Medicine and Biosciences, College of Osteopathic Medicine in 1983. She served her internship at the University Hospital in Kansas City, Missouri, and her internal medicine residency at the University of Missouri Kansas City School of Medicine, where she also had a fellowship in pulmonary diseases and critical care medicine in 1989.

In addition to her research credentials, Dr. Willsie has had an exceptional career in academic medicine. She rapidly worked her way up the academic and administrative ladders at both University of Missouri Kansas City School of Medicine and Kansas City University of Medicine and Biosciences, College of Osteopathic Medicine. She was assistant dean for first- and second-year studies, interim chair of the Department of Medicine, and professor of medicine at University of Missouri Kansas City School of Medicine. At present she is executive vice president for academic affairs/dean at Kansas City University of Medicine and Biosciences, College of Osteopathic Medicine.

Dr. Willsie has received numerous awards and honors. She was given the Young Investigator Award by the American College of Chest Physicians and the Researcher of the Year award by the American College of Osteopathic Internists. She was placed in the Mentor Hall of Fame by the AOA and received the Meritorious Alumni Achievement Award from Pittsburg State University, just to name a few.[33] Dr. Willsie is also a member of the Anesthesia and Respiratory Therapy Devices Panel of the US Food and Drug Administration.[34]

Denise K. Burns, DO

Denise Burns graduated from the University of New England, College of Osteopathic Medicine in 1993. While still an undergraduate student at the State University of New York, she was named American Chemistry Student of the Year. She served her internship and residency in family practice at St. Barnabas Hospital in Far Rockaway, New York, where she was named Family Practice Resident of the Year.

As of spring 2011, Dr. Burns is residency director of family practice at the Southampton Hospital; she was previously an associate professor of osteopathic manipulative medicine at the Philadelphia College of Osteopathic Medicine and before that, served on the faculty of the New York College of Osteopathic Medicine. She is a practicing physician at the Academic Health Center at Philadelphia College of Osteopathic Medicine and maintains a private practice in Syosset, New York. She has hospital affiliations with Long Beach Medical Center and St. John's Episcopal Hospital in New York.

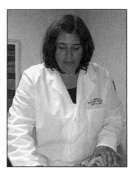

Denise E. Burns, DO

Research by faculty members at colleges of osteopathic medicine has become an increasingly important part of academic activities in recent years. Dr. Burns has conducted research on:

- The effects of OMT on cardiac arrhythmias and on hypothyroidism
- Radioactive isotope usage and breast carcinoma detection
- Effects of osteopathic muscle energy techniques on cervical spine motion
- High-velocity low-amplitude quantitative force study
- Parkinson's disease and effectiveness of OMT[35]

Karen T. Snider, DO

Even before graduating from the West Virginia School of Osteopathic Medicine in 1998, Karen Snider began her career in osteopathic research. After completing her internship at Greenbrier Valley Medical Center in Ronceverte, West Virginia, Dr. Snider served her residency in osteopathic neuromusculoskeletal medicine at Northeast Regional Medical Center in Kirksville, Missouri. She is currently director of Undergraduate Osteopathic Manipulative Medicine Fellows, as well as associate professor in the department of neuromusculoskeletal medicine at the A. T. Still University of Health Sciences, Kirksville College of Osteopathic Medicine.

Dr. Snider has an impressive list of research projects including:

- Beta-adrenergic receptor site changes and vasodilatation ability of rats fed the repartitioning agent L644, 969
- Effects of OMT on childhood otitis media outcomes
- Interexaminer reliability of osteopathic palpatory evaluation of the lumbar spine
- Evaluation of the relationship between impaired vertebral mobility and bone mineral density

- Interexaminer reliability of osteopathic palpatory examinations
- Effects of OMT on bone density
- Use of skin markers to identify the spinous processes of L1 to L4

- Measuring of the interexaminer reliability of tests commonly used in the osteopathic profession to evaluate somatic dysfunction

Dr. Snider has an equally impressive list of medical publications. She is board certified in osteopathic neuromusculoskeletal medicine. As of spring 2011, Dr. Snider is chair of the department of manipulative medicine at A. T. Still University, Kirksville College of Osteopathic Medicine, and is on the staff of Northeast Regional Medical Center in Kirksville, Missouri.[36]

Kendi Hensel, DO/PhD

Postdoctoral programs that train DO/PhD researchers are no longer a luxury for the profession but a necessity. After graduating from Louisiana Scholars' College at Northwestern State University, Kendi Hensel received her DO degree from the Oklahoma State University, College of Osteopathic Medicine in 1998, and her PhD from the University of North Texas Health Science Center in 2009. She also completed a post-doctoral fellowship in osteopathic manipulative medicine clinical research and education.

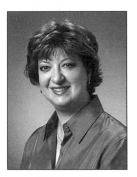

Kendi Hensel, DO

Dr. Hensel's list of accomplishments and awards is already impressive, and she has a significant list of research publications and grants to her name. As of spring 2011, Dr. Hensel is an associate professor of osteopathic manipulative medicine at University of North Texas Health Science Center.[37]

NOTES

1. See Still, *Autobiography*; and Trowbridge, *Andrew Taylor Still*, esp. 94–129, 134–40.
2. Walter, *First School of Osteopathic Medicine*, 80; and "Beginning of the Research Movement," *Osteopathic Physician* 14 (Dec. 1908): 11–12.
3. Dr. Smith's article was reproduced in the *Journal of Osteopathy* 5, no. 8 (Jan. 1899). See also Grigg, "Peripatetic Pioneer: William Smith, MD, DO (1862–1912)," *Journal of the History of Medicine* 22 (Apr. 1967): 169–79.
4. Walter, *First School of Osteopathic Medicine*, 79–80.
5. Wright, *Perspectives in Osteopathic Medicine*, 18–19; and Gevitz, *The DOs*, 62.
6. Gevitz, *The DOs*, 62–63; and Burns, "Woman's Osteopathic Club Builds House for the A. T. Still Research Institute," *Western Osteopath* (May 1925): 16.
7. "College Recommended for Federal Grant," *Journal of Osteopathy* 54 (Jan. 1947): 21–22.

8. Osteopathic Research Center, *ORC Annual Report, 2008–09*; and Osteopathic Research Center, "Mission and Goals," accessed 30 April 2008, www.hsc.unt.edu/orc.

9. Crosby, *Epidemic and Peace*, 206–7.

10. "Osteopathy's Epidemic Record," *Osteopathic Physician* 36, no. 1 (July 1919): 1; and Riley, "Osteopathy's Power over Flu-Pneumonia," *Osteopathic Physician* 36, no. 1 (July 1919): 6.

11. Reed, "Prevention and Treatment of Influenza," *JAOA* 18 1 (1919): 209–11; and Quinn and Byrne, "Physician," 478.

12. Allison, "My Impression of the Flu," *Journal of Osteopathy* 26, no. 7 (July 1919): 289–91.

13. Tucker, "Spanish Influenza: What and Why," *JAOA* 18, no. 6 (Feb. 1919): 270–73.

14. Allison, "My Impression of the Flu," *Journal of Osteopathy* 26, no. 7 (July 1919): 290.

15. Hodge et al., "Lymphatic Pump Treatment Increases Leukocyte Numbers in Thoracic Duct Lymph," *JAOA* 106, no. 8 (Aug. 2006): 496.

16. Booth, *History of Osteopathy*, 387–89.

17. See Abrams, *New Concepts in Diagnosis and Treatment*, esp. 337–73.

18. Armstrong and Armstrong, *Great American Medicine Show*, 192–94; and Walter, *First School of Osteopathic Medicine*, 140.

19. Armstrong and Armstrong, *Great American Medicine Show*, 193; and "What ERA Means to Osteopaths," *Achievement* 2 (April 1923): 5–10.

20. Walter, *First School of Osteopathic Medicine*, 140; and Armstrong and Armstrong, *Great American Medicine Show*, 192–94.

21. Gevitz, *The DOs*, 184–86.

22. Heath and Gevitz, "Research Status of Somatic Dysfunction," 1188, 1193.

23. Andersson et al., "Comparison of Osteopathic Spinal Manipulation with Standard Care for Patients with Low Back Pain," *New England Journal of Medicine* 341, no. 19 (Nov. 1999): 1426–31.

24. DO/PhD programs are available at Michigan State University, College of Osteopathic Medicine; Ohio University, College of Osteopathic Medicine; Oklahoma State University, College of Osteopathic Medicine; Philadelphia College of Osteopathic Medicine; University of Medicine and Dentistry of New Jersey, College of Osteopathic Medicine; and University of North Texas Health Science Center, Texas College of Osteopathic Medicine.

25. Beal, "Foreword," *American Academy of Osteopathy Yearbook* (1994): iv.

26. Fitzgerald, "Women in History, Pioneers of the Profession," *The DO* 25 (1984): 70–71.

27. DiGiovanna, *Encyclopedia of Osteopathy*, 103.

28. College of Osteopathic Physicians and Surgeons, *Western Alumnus of the College of Osteopathic Physicians and Surgeons,* directory for June 1935.

29. Perloff, *To Secure Merit*, 32.

30. Miriam Mills, MD, personal correspondence with the author, 5 December 2006.

31. Karen Steele, DO, personal correspondence with the author, 5 December 2006 and 12 February 2011.

32. Terrie Taylor, DO, personal correspondence with the author, 27 November 2006; and *AOA Newsletter*, 9 February 2011.

33. Sandra Willsie, DO, personal correspondence with the author, 19 December 2006.

34. *AOA Daily Report*, 21 April 2009, 1.

35. Denise Burns, DO, personal correspondence with the author, 8 June 2007 and 26 January 2011.

36. Karen Snider, DO, personal correspondence with the author, 5 January 2007.

37. Kendi Hensel, DO, personal correspondence with the author, 13 April 2007.

Chapter Seven

Women Osteopathic Physicians in the Uniformed Services

"I began to see, during the Civil War, in those portions of the states of Missouri and Kansas where the doctors were shut out, the children did not die."

Andrew Taylor Still, MD, DO

"I have given to women a chance. The lily of hope has come to the bed of anguish."

Andrew Taylor Still, MD, DO

As a young man, Andrew Taylor Still served the Union cause as a physician in the Kansas militia (see pp. 20–21). Later, when he opened the first osteopathic college, he named the school for his beloved country. Given Dr. Still's military record and his dedication to providing medical care for soldiers, it is ironic that one of the greatest struggles the osteopathic profession has endured was the fight to gain acceptance for osteopathic physicians who wished to serve as medical officers in the armed services. And that struggle is itself ironic because one of the early successes that brought public attention to osteopathy involved soldiers.

The following article, titled "A Soldier's Story from the Spanish American War," was published in the October 1898 *Journal of Osteopathy*.

A passenger train from the east was thundering along over the steel rails bearing many travelers to the great and glorious west. At a point in the eastern border of Ohio the train stopped to make connection from New York, which brought two Santiago heroes. Every eye was strained to catch a glimpse of the boys in blue as they came on board, pale, emaciated, and only wrecks of the former strong healthy young men who in the spring time marched away in health and buoyancy.

145

But their cheeks, wan and sunken were flushed with fever. The passengers and conductor freely offered them the best on the train. As no berths could be obtained for them, two ladies on the sleeper gave up their berths to the heroes, one of whom had been at the storming of El Caney, and the other at San Juan heights where he lay nine days in the trenches before Santiago. Alternately soaked by drenching rains, and parched by tropical suns, no wonder he was fever stricken.

The conductor soon discovered he had two seriously ill aboard. Their temperature was 104 and their pulses had reached the danger point. He telegraphed to the next stopping point, "Have physician at depot. Sick soldiers aboard."

Physicians and ladies with all dainties possible were at hand, but alas the poor heroes could not enjoy them. They lay in their berths with raging fevers. The doctors administered their doses but without any effect—they grew worse.

At last a lady asked to be permitted to try her skill at reducing the fever. She gave the patient some cracked ice, threw the doctor's medicine out of the car window, sat at the patient's side and slipping her hand under his head began some mysterious movements along his neck and spine. In a short time respiration became more easy, his temperature was reduced, and his pulse grew normal, his fever was gone and he slept like a baby. To the next soldier she hastened. Here was a more serious case than the first. He had had yellow fever and was suffering with his spine. The young lady at once began operating on his spine and neck. Under the magical touch of his mysterious unknown friend the fever was quickly reduced and it was gone and he too slept like a baby.

"How did you do that?"

"It is a miracle."

"Who are you?"

"What strange power do you have that you can heal the sick at a touch?"

These and a hundred similar questions were asked, she answered: "Bless me not, but the science of Osteopathy."

All night long the soldiers slept and next morning when they came to change cars each was able to walk away with their grips in their hands. One of the soldiers was private Charles Pratt of Springfield Illinois; the other was from Fort Worth, Texas; both of the regular army.

The young lady who accomplished the wonderful care and no doubt saved the lives of the heroes of Santiago, was Miss Julia L. Hart, of Clarksburg, West Virginia, a student in A. T. Still's American School of Osteopathy. Miss Hart declares that the gratification she felt on relieving those sick heroes amply repaid her for all her long months of hard study. What higher accomplishment need a lady ask than to be an Osteopath?[1]

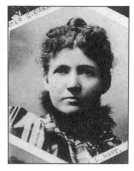

Julia L. Hart
[detail, 1899 ASO graduation picture, MOM]

This young osteopathic medical student did nothing magical; she simply used logic and her osteopathic training. Instead of using the ineffective drugs notorious in that era, Julia Hart gave the soldiers ice chips to help to reduce their fever and replace much-needed fluids. The story is vague as to the specific osteopathic treatment that was given and tells only that the student worked on the soldiers' spines and necks. If she used standard osteopathic treatments of the era, she would have worked with the sympathetic nerves that arise from the ganglia (nerve bundles) located just lateral to the thoracic and upper lumbar spines; these nerves go to the blood vessels and sweat glands of the skin and cause peripheral vasodilatation (enlarging of the blood vessels in the skin), which increases the loss of body heat through the skin.[2] Then working with the neck and collar area, she would have relaxed the muscles and fascia (connective tissue) that would have released any restrictions to the blood and lymphatic flow through the thoracic outlet (outlet of the chest cage).[3] There osteopathic manipulative treatments have been proven to increase the release of disease-fighting white blood cells into the circulating blood.[4] Although this extrapolation from details of the story seems tantalizingly corroborative, there is insufficient information to know definitively which treatments Hart provided; however, it can be assumed that Hart abided by the basic tenets of osteopathy in treating the soldiers. She addressed the needs of the whole person by soothing the patients and attending to their psychological stresses, in this case using the *feminine touch*. And, not least of all, she worked with the soldiers to assist their bodies' self-healing mechanisms. When they awoke they were not cured, but their homeostatic capabilities were greatly improved and their bodies had started on the pathway to recovery. While some details can be gleaned from this account, the statement that she "threw the doctor's medicine out the car window" may be attributed to the propensity of nineteenth-century prose for hyperbole, but does emphasize the fact that Miss Hart achieved success without the use of drugs.

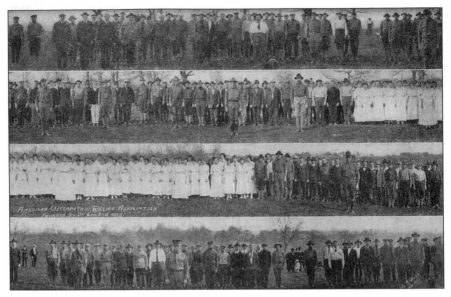

The American Osteopathic Relief Association founded 13 April 1917. This is a compressed version of a 10 foot panoramic picture taken on 13 May 1917, the first time the AORA lined up in a regimental formation. [July 1917 *JAOA*, p. 278, MOM]

The first great need for physicians to treat sick or wounded soldiers after the founding of the osteopathic profession came with the outbreak of World War I. Osteopathic physicians, like most patriotic Americans, lined up to help their country by enlisting in the military services. The military, however, rejected the DOs as physicians;[5] the American Red Cross also rejected DOs as physicians. It was not until 1952 that the American Red Cross finally recognized DOs.[6]

Not to be denied the opportunity to serve their country as physicians, George Still, DO, the great nephew of A. T. Still and surgeon in chief of the Hospital of the American School of Osteopathy, organized the American Osteopathic Relief Association (AORA), which was composed of the attending physicians, nurses, student nurses, and staff of the osteopathic hospital, as well as the faculty and medical students of the American School of Osteopathy.[7] The AORA was modeled after the American Red Cross and performed similar functions. The AORA conducted educational instruction on such subjects as army hygiene, camp sanitation, and care of wounds received in battle. Classes were taught by the faculty of the osteopathic medical school and members of the Missouri National Guard. The newest methods of combat first aid were taught, and training was given on the system of medical care being used on the battlefields of Europe.

Dr. George Still was named the organization's director general and the AORA was organized into a regiment consisting of two battalions. Each battalion was comprised of three companies of fifty persons each. Col. George Still, DO, was the regimental commander and Lieut. Col. Charles Still, DO, the son of Andrew T. Still, was the executive officer. Women as well as men participated in this patriotic war effort.[8] Each member wore on their left arm an armband with the emblem of the AORA, which consisted of a white cross on a blue background.

The AORA applied for official government recognition as a relief organization to function similarly to the American Red Cross, and although recognition never came, the AORA continued to function for the duration of the war. The organization struggled to retain their strength of numbers as many members were drafted into the armed services.[9] Many DOs used their medical training as medics and corpsmen in the Medical Service Corps but were never officially recognized as physicians. During World War I, neither being an osteopathic physician, an osteopathic medical student, or a member of AORA was recognized by the draft board as a reason for a deferment.

WOMEN OSTEOPATHIC PHYSICIANS DURING WORLD WAR I

Despite being unable to serve as physicians in the military or the American Red Cross, some osteopathic physicians found other ways to serve. Bessie Srofe, DO, joined the Salvation Army and in the course of her duties, was sent to the front lines in France. Although her duties were not officially those of a physician, she received permission from the Salvation Army Headquarters stating that since she was the only professional woman with the Salvation Army, "[she] should render professional services so long as you do not antagonize the Red Cross or army doctors." She was first assigned to Field Hospital No. 148, where she provided physician services to American soldiers. She was especially pleased with this assignment because she was caring for soldiers from the Thirty-Seventh Division from her home state of Ohio. Over the course of her six-month assignment in France, Dr. Srofe was assigned to three different field hospitals and frequently assisted in surgery. Speaking of her experience in France during the war, Dr. Srofe stated, "I have gained professionally as there was not a day I did not render professional service."[10]

Another osteopathic physician, Jane Wells Craven of Pittsburgh, Pennsylvania, raised funds and took the Pittsburgh field ambulance and ambulance crew to France

where they joined the French Hospital Service. Dr.
Craven served as a surgeon in French hospitals and
frequently performed surgery while under bom-
bardment from German forces. Several of her
American companions from the ambulance crew
were killed in enemy attacks. The French government decorated Jane Craven with the Croix
de Guerre (Cross of War) for bravery under fire
and devotion to duty. She was the first American
woman to ever receive this distinguished honor.[11]

On 20 June 1917, bill HR 5118 was submitted to the House of Representatives allowing
for the commissioning of osteopathic physicians
into the US Armed Services on an equal basis
with MDs;[12] unfortunately this bill did not pass.
Then a next attempt, bill HR 5407, was approved
and signed into law to "provide for the selection
of osteopathic physicians in the medical service of
the Army and Navy."[13] The bill provided for the
DOs to have "the same official status, rank, pay,
and allowance of officers of corresponding grade
in the medical service."[14] The DOs were required
to be fully licensed in the state where they practiced and to take an examination. Twenty-five
fully licensed DOs took the examination for the

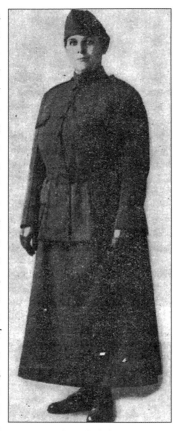

Bessie Srofe, DO
[1919 *Journal of Osteopathy*, MOM]

Army; the first fifteen all passed, and the scores of the remaining ten DOs were
never released,[15] though it is probable that they also all passed. Regardless, Army
Surgeon General William Gorgas, MD, a past American Medical Society (AMA)
president, would not give commissions to these DOs. This occurred during a time
when the US Army physician shortage was so dire that the surgeon general was
giving commissions to homeopathic physicians and allopathic physicians who had
graduated from non-AMA approved medical schools, as long as they could pass
an examination.[16] Gorgas continued to deny medical commissions to osteopathic
physicians, citing the Flexner Report of 1910 as the basis for his decision.[17]

The American Osteopathic Association (AOA) and the osteopathic physicians mounted a national public relations blitz. Tens of thousands of supporters sent
letters to legislators asking them to commission DOs in the military. One of these

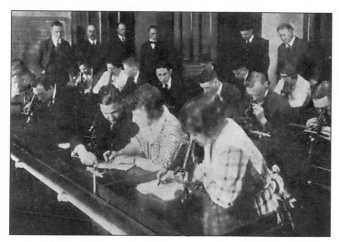

Microbiology laboratory at the Philadelphia College of Osteopathy, 1920. [PCO Announcement, 1920–1921, PCOM]

letters came from former president Theodore Roosevelt. Unfortunately, Congress failed to act on his request.[18]

Following World War I, the osteopathic profession and the AOA did not continue to press for equality in the military. During the war, most DOs had expanded their practices, and combined with the publicity the profession had received following their successes in fighting the influenza epidemic of 1918/19, most DOs were content to maintain the status quo.[19] This was a mistake that the profession would long regret. It was another fifty years before DOs were finally commissioned as medical officers on an equal basis with MDs.

After World War I, female enrollment at osteopathic hospitals declined from 50 percent in 1923 to just over 10 percent in 1938. This decline continued until the start of World War II. Soldiers returning from war and enrolling in medical school was one reason for this decline, but perhaps more importantly, during the Depression of the 1930s, families had less money to spend on education and chose to use their limited funds to educate sons rather than daughters. Female physicians and medical students felt that gender discrimination was also a major factor.[20]

Between the two world wars, there were some minor advancements in the recognition of DOs by the federal government. In 1929, the US Congress passed legislation that made DOs and MDs equal for licensure in the District of Columbia, and in 1938 DOs were recognized as physicians for the purpose of the Federal Compensation Act. In 1940, as a result of lobbying by the AOA, medical students attending osteopathic medical colleges were given deferments from military service until graduation.[21] The Military (Army) Appropriations Act was approved by Congress on 30 June 1941 and signed into law by President Franklin D. Roosevelt. It provided for "the pay of internes [*sic*] who are graduates of or have successfully completed at least four years professional training in reputable schools of medicine or osteopathy…"[22] Following the attack on Pearl Harbor on 7 December 1941, many osteopathic physicians tried to enlist in the military; however, they continued to be rejected as physicians. Most DOs who enlisted in the army were used as medics or placed in other medically related areas. Quintus Drennan, DO (ASO 1916), for example, was placed in charge of corrective work and casting at the Walter Reed Army Hospital in Washington, DC.[23]

The Navy Appropriations Act approved by Congress on 26 October 1942 and signed by President Roosevelt provided for "the pay of commissioned medical officers who are graduates of reputable schools of osteopathy." Unfortunately the bill also contained the qualification that DOs were to be commissioned "as may be determined and approved by the Secretary of the Navy."[24] The Secretary of the Navy never approved a single DO and none were ever commissioned. Osteopathic physicians in the Navy during World War II were classified as pharmacist mates second class, instead of medical officers as intended by Congress and the president, and MDs were able to maintain control of the medical corps in all branches of the US military.

Following the war, Public Law 604 passed in 1946, again authorizing the commissioning of DOs as medical officers. Because of pressure from the AMA, threatening to withdraw its approval from military hospitals and force closure of military postgraduate training programs, the Truman administration failed to act on this authority. Once again the AMA used its power to deprive the osteopathic profession. Many returning servicemen and women used funds available through the GI Bill to attend osteopathic medical schools;[25] however, these fully licensed osteopathic physicians and surgeons were still denied commissions as medical officers in the armed services. The paradox was that any DO who had attended an osteopathic medical school on the GI Bill could not use that taxpayer-funded medical education to again serve their country as a medical officer in the military. This absurdity continued until 1967.

In late 1945, the Veterans Administration announced that osteopathic physicians would be accepted for appointments to the Department of Medicine and Surgery. The administration indicated that any appointee to the Department of Medicine and Surgery must "hold the degree of doctor of medicine or doctor of osteopathy from a college or university approved by the administrator and have completed an internship satisfactory to the administrator and be licensed to practice medicine in one of the states or territories of the United States." It took over a year to take all the steps required, but by 1947 all six of the existing osteopathic colleges and fifty-four osteopathic hospitals had met the needed requirements. On 5 May 1947, the first DO began treating patients in the Veterans Administration. The Veterans Administration also gave osteopathic hospitals clearance to treat disabled veterans in emergencies when no veterans' facilities were available.[26]

In October 1953, Dr. Murray Goldstein became the first DO to be commissioned as a medical officer by the US Public Health Service.[27] In 1995, Joyce M. Johnson, DO, became the first female DO to be appointed an admiral in the US Public Health Service. She went on to become the first woman chief medical officer for the US Coast Guard.[28]

Finally, in March 1956, the osteopaths got the legislation they had been seeking for so many years—or so they thought! The US Congress passed HR 483 and the act was signed by President Dwight D. Eisenhower. The act stated that any qualified graduate of an accredited osteopathic medical school, upon acceptance into the uniformed services must receive his/her commission as a medical officer, equivalent to an allopathic physician.[29] The AMA and the surgeons general of all branches of the armed forces vigorously opposed this act, and unfortunately, the wording of this act again allowed a loophole. The all-MD military medical hierarchy defied the law and simply refused to accept DOs into the military service so they would not have to give them medical commissions. A difference in opinion as to how to handle this issue that developed between the California Osteopathic Association and the AOA was one of the multiple precipitating causes of the civil war within the osteopathic profession of 1958 to 1962.[30]

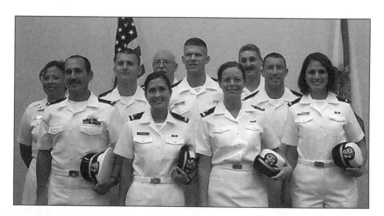

Commissioning ceremony for US Navy scholarship recipients, 12 August 2005, LECOM, Bradenton. Left to right: Randal Scott, Paul Bures, Prudence Knigge, Keith Knigge, Rachel Sanchez, Daniel Heard, and Aidth Flores. [Lisa Cambridge and LECOM, Bradenton]

In 1966, the Vietnam War was increasing in intensity and the armed services found themselves facing a shortage of medical officers. The war was very unpopular and the dwindling number of volunteer MDs could not keep pace with the demand for physicians. This military physician shortage made it necessary for President Lyndon B. Johnson to declare the need for the first physician draft since World War II,[31] and the military medical establishment was prepared to again refuse commissions to DOs despite the executive order.

It was the unpopularity of the Vietnam War that accounted for the shortage of physicians in the first place, and that was also the reason MDs were outraged that they were being drafted and DOs were being excluded. The Camden County, New Jersey, Medical Society asked their congressman to speak to the House of Representatives about this issue. He reported to Congress that both the MDs and the DOs in his district opposed the AMA opposition to DOs being included in the draft. As a result, congressional pressure was placed on Secretary of Defense Robert McNamara, who then, invoking the 1956 law (HR 483), ordered the surgeons general of all branches of the military services to accept osteopathic physicians as fully accredited physicians and surgeons in the military services.[32] This was the last step needed for DOs to finally become commissioned medical officers in the US military. Because of Secretary McNamara's order, the surgeons general had no option but to draft both DOs and MDs, and 111 DOs were drafted. In 1967, these DOs, along with a small number of volunteers, were taken into the armed forces as the first commissioned osteopathic medical officers, and the fifty-year struggle had ended. Today osteopathic physicians serve with pride and distinction as commissioned medical officers in all branches of the US Military and Public Health Services and are recognized as physicians by the American Red Cross. Lt. Gen. Ronald Blank, DO, achieved the highest rank of any physician in the military when he became the first osteopathic physician to serve as the surgeon general of the US Army.[33] Military and Public Health Service scholarships are equally available to osteopathic and allopathic medical students. The draft rules were changed in 1968, making the graduates from that year the first osteopathic medical students to be deferred from a military draft until the completion of their internship and/or residency.[34]

Joyce M. Johnson, DO
Joyce M. Johnson, DO, MA, has many firsts in the osteopathic profession related to her service in the of the US Public Health Service Commissioned Corps. While still a student at Michigan State University College of Osteopathic Medicine, she

was the first osteopathic medical student to do a rotation at the Centers for Disease Control and Prevention (CDC). Upon receiving her DO degree in 1980, she was commissioned into the US Public Health Service Commissioned Corps. After completing a rotating internship, she was the first DO to serve in the CDC's prestigious Epidemiologic Intelligence Officer Program, and was among the first AIDS research-

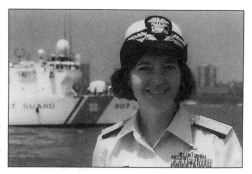

Rear Admiral (ret.) Joyce M. Johnson, DO, MA; USPHS [James A. Calderwood Jr.]

ers. She was the first DO to complete the CDC's Public Health and Preventive Medicine residency. Dr. Johnson was in the first group of DOs to take the osteopathic public health and preventive medicine specialty board examinations. She later served on the boards of the American Osteopathic College of Public Health and Preventive Medicine and the corresponding American Osteopathic Board of Public Health and Preventive Medicine.

Dr. Johnson's career in the US Public Health Service spanned nearly twenty-four years with assignments to several other agencies, including the Bureau of Hospitals and Clinics, US Food and Drug Administration, National Institute of Mental Health, and Substance Abuse and Mental Health Services Administration. In 1995, she was promoted to rear admiral lower half (one-star admiral) and was the first female osteopathic physician to achieve that rank. In 1997, she was appointed director of health and safety and chief medical officer of the US Coast Guard. In this position she functioned as the coast guard's surgeon general and was the first female flag officer in coast guard uniform. Records suggest this also made her the first female physician, DO or MD, to serve as a flag or general officer with any military service. Dr. Johnson received her second star shortly after being assigned to the US Coast Guard. She was the first woman and the first DO to serve on the Board of Trustees of the US Coast Guard Academy.

Dr. Johnson has received five honorary doctoral degrees from osteopathic colleges and universities and is board certified in three specialties: public health/preventive medicine, psychiatry, and clinical pharmacology. In addition, she is a certified addiction specialist and a certified food service executive. Prior to her commissioning, she earned a master's degree in hospital and health administration.

Dr. Johnson has also received over forty awards and ribbons, including a Distinguished Service Medal and two Outstanding Service Medals (one with valor). She has over sixty publications and writes several regular columns. She has lectured throughout the world and has extensive international health experience on all seven continents. She has been part of many on-site disaster response teams, and was the first DO on a Disaster Medical Assistance Team, serving from 1985 to 2003. Since that time, she has volunteered with DOCARE, Project HOPE, and others. Rear Admiral Johnson is active with the Uniformed Services University of Health Sciences and the Georgetown University Medical Schools. She was also the first woman and first osteopathic physician to serve on the US Coast Guard Board of Trustees. She retired from the US Public Health Service with the rank of rear admiral upper half (two-star admiral) and was appointed vice president of health sciences, Battelle Memorial Institute in December 2003. [35]

Gail Fancher, DO

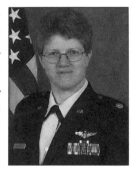

Lt. Col. Fancher began her military career serving as a US Air Force nurse for four years; she transferred to the Air Force Reserves while attending medical school. After graduating from the University of Health Sciences College of Osteopathic Medicine in Kansas City, Missouri, in 1984, Dr. Fancher completed a surgical internship at Kessler Medical Center, Kessler Air Force Base, Mississippi, after which she started her professional career as a flight surgeon. She is board certified in family practice, osteopathic manipulative medicine, and aerospace medicine.

Lt. Col. Gail Fancher, DO, US Air Force Medical Corps

Lt. Col. Gail D. Fancher is the Ninety-Seventh Medical Group chief of aerospace medicine. She ensures crews are physically ready to fly advanced military aircraft worth $5.95 billion. She has a passion for aerospace evacuation and has served as validating flight surgeon at Scott Air Force Base and in Qatar. Dr. Fancher has been deployed four times and redeployed three more times, the most recent as Mobile Aeromedical Staging Facility flight surgeon in Kuwait City. [36]

Mimms J. Mabee, DO, MPH

Col. Mabee obtained her bachelor's and master's degrees from California State University in Los Angeles. She received her DO degree from the Kirksville College of Osteopathic Medicine in 1986 and served her rotating internship in Kirksville, Missouri. In 1987, she joined the US Army as a general medical officer, serving at the Aberdeen Proving Grounds until 1990 when she returned to civilian life to pursue specialty training in occupational medicine. She received her master's in public health at the Medical College of Wisconsin. Dr. Mabee became board certified in occupational and environmental medicine in 1998. During her time in civilian practice, she remained active in the US Army Reserve. In 2003, she was recalled to active duty and served as the acting chief of preventive medicine at Fort Campbell,

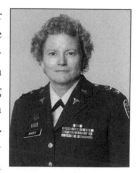

Col. Mimms J. Mabee, DO, MPH, US Army Medical Corps

Kentucky, before being deployed to Iraq. Upon her return from the war zone, Dr. Mabee decided to remain on full-time active duty in the army.

Col. Mabee is an expert on chemical, biological, radiological, nuclear, and explosive devices, and has served two tours in Iraq. As of spring 2011, she is chief of preventive medicine at Barquist Army Health Clinic at Fort Detrick, Maryland, which includes duty as the biosecurity chief at the US Army Research Institute of Infectious Disease.[37]

NOTES

1. Still, "A Soldier's Story," *Journal of Osteopathy* 5, no. 5 (Oct. 1898): 246–47.

2. Ward, *Foundations for Osteopathic Medicine*, 97–98.

3. DiGiovanna and Schiowitz, *Osteopathic Approach to Diagnosis and Treatment* (1991), 436–37.

4. Hodge et al., "Lymphatic Pump Treatment Increases Leukocyte Numbers in Thoracic Duct Lymph," *JAOA* 106, no. 8 (Aug. 2006): 496.

5. Riley, "Professional Duty and Opportunity," *JAOA* 17 (Aug. 1918): 654–62.

6. "Red Cross Authorized DOs," *Forum of Osteopathy* 26 (Oct. 1952): 201–2.

7. "American Osteopathic Relief Association," *Journal of Osteopathy* 24 (May 1917): 278–84.

8. Ibid.

9. Ibid.

10. Srofe, "Osteopath in Salvation Army over There," *Journal of Osteopathy* 26, no. 3 (March 1919): 145–48.

11. "News of the Month," *Journal of Osteopathy* 25, no. 2 (Feb. 1918): 101.

12. HR 5118, 65th Cong., 1st sess. (June 20, 1917) 1–2.

13. HR 5407, 65th Cong., 1st sess. (1917) 1–2.

14. Gevitz, "Sword and the Scalpel," 279–80.

15. Riley, "Professional Duty and Opportunity," *JAOA* 17 (Aug, 1918): 854–62.

16. Gevitz, "Sword and the Scalpel," 280.

17. Ibid.

18. DiGiovanna and Schiowitz, *Osteopathic Approach to Diagnosis and Treatment*, 8.

19. Gevitz, "Sword and the Scalpel," 281–82.

20. Walter, *Women and Osteopathic Medicine*, 20–21.

21. Gevitz, "Sword and the Scalpel," 282.

22. Pub. L. No. 139, 55 Stat. 300 (1941).

23. "Dr. Drennan Teaching Plaster Work," *Journal of Osteopathy* 26 (May 1919): 252.

24. Pub. L. No. 763, 55 Stat. 366 (1942) sec. 102.

25. Gevitz, "Sword and Scalpel," 283.

26. "Veterans' Administration," *Journal of Osteopathy* 54, no. 1 (Jan. 1947): 25; and "Appointed to Veterans' Administration," *Journal of Osteopathy* 54, no. 5 (May 1947): 28.

27. Tilley, "Osteopathic Education," *Forum of Osteopathy* 25 (Apr. 1951): 23.

28. Burnett, "Women Contribute Greatly to Medicine: Andrew Taylor Still Memorial Address," *The DO* (Oct. 1999): 56.

29. *Appointment of Doctors of Osteopathy as Medical Officers. Hearings on HR 483 Before a Subcommittee of the Committee on Armed Services*, US Senate, 84th Cong., 2nd sess., 14 February and 2 March 1956.

30. Gevitz, "Sword and the Scalpel," 282–83.

31. Exec. Order No. 11266, Fed. Reg. 743 (20 Jan. 1966).

32. Gevitz, "Sword and the Scalpel," 284.

33. Perloff, *To Secure Merit*, 91.

34. Walter, *First School of Osteopathic Medicine*, 402.

35. Joyce Johnson, personal correspondence with the author, 12 May 2008.

36. Gail Fancher, personal correspondence with the author, 19 March 2007.

37. Mimms J. Mabee, personal correspondence with the author, 28 March 2008.

Chapter Eight

Osteopathic Nurses

"Woman is finer principled than man, she is sensory, man motor. He is motor, she is intellectual."

Andrew Taylor Still, MD, DO

"Women are especially adapted for osteopathic work as they are sympathetic, cheerful, courageous and hopeful, characteristics which are greatly to be desired."

Ella Still, DO

THE NEED FOR OSTEOPATHICALLY TRAINED nurses became immediately apparent with the opening of the first osteopathic hospital. So the American School of Osteopathy (ASO) Hospital initiated an osteopathic nursing school that opened in 1906, just months following the opening of the hospital itself. Leone Dalton, an ASO medical student, was the first director of the ASO Training School for Nurses. The purpose of the school was to train nurses based on the new science of osteopathy, since nurses prior to the opening of this school had been trained in allopathic hospitals and did not understand osteopathic principles and practice. The second director of the ASO nursing school was Mary Walters, RN, DO.[1] Dr. Walters strove to improve the training of nurses in the new osteopathic

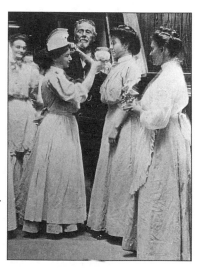

Dr. A. T. Still instructing student nurses in the operating room of the ASO Hospital, ca. 1908.
[MOM PH 1077a(2)]

hospital so she traveled to Minnesota and inspected the Mayo hospital. She then based the training of the osteopathic nurses on the training methods she had observed in the nurse training program at the Mayo hospital.[2]

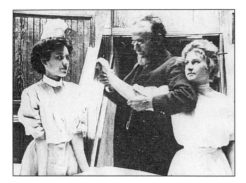

The "Old Doctor," Dr. A.T. Still demonstrating manipulative techniques to student nurses at the ASO Hospital, ca. 1908. [MOM PH 1493]

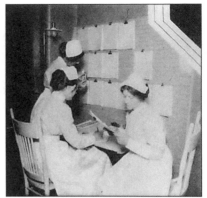

Nurses Station, ASO hospital, 1915. Note the single bare bulb as the only source of light. [MOM 2006.20.04]

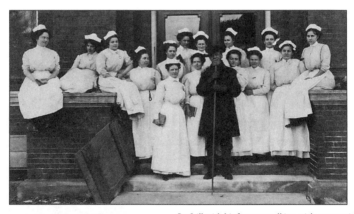

Dr. Still with his famous walking stick, poses with student nurses on the front steps of the American School of Osteopathy Hospital, 1910–11. [MOM PH 894]

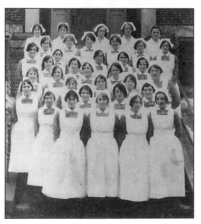

Student nurses outside of Laughlin Osteopathic Hospital, Kirksville, MO, ca. 1929. [MOM 2006.20.05]

The Laughlin Training School for Nurses opened in August 1919 as an adjunct to the Laughlin Osteopathic Hospital, which had opened in 1918. A large house adjacent to the hospital located on the site of A. T. Still's old home was obtained for the nurses' residence. Ruth Story, RN, was the director at the time. Concerns that the opening of the Laughlin Osteopathic Hospital across the street from the ASO Hospital would adversely influence the occupancy rate of either hospital were soon put to rest. Both hospitals were soon functioning at full capacity and the need for additional facilities became very quickly apparent. With the ASO Hospital unable to accommodate additional patients, the school opened two specialty hospitals during 1918. The nurses' quarters on the corner of Osteopathy and Jefferson Streets was converted into an eye, ear, nose, and throat specialty hospital, which led to the expansion of that department and the addition of a course in ophthalmoscopy and refraction to the fourth-year medical school curriculum. Later the same year, the ASO, still short of hospital beds, attempted to purchase the local MD hospital, the Grim Medical Hospital, without success.[3] The ASO then purchased a large residence and converted it into the Missouri Woman's Hospital, which opened in October 1918 to provide additional obstetrics and gynecology hospital facilities. The ASO medical and nursing students also received training in these specialty hospitals. From 1919 until 1925, the two osteopathic nursing schools operated separately just across the street from each other. In 1925, they merged when the ASO and the A. T. Still College of Osteopathy also came together. Ruth Story continued to direct the combined nursing schools as superintendent. The nursing school continued to train high-quality nurses until it closed in 1949.[4]

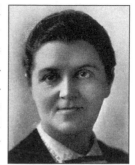

Ruth Ann Story, RN
[1943 *Osteoblast*, MOM]

Nelda Martin Richardson, RN, and Louise Martin Warren, RN

Sisters Louise and Nelda Martin studied osteopathic nursing at the Laughlin Osteopathic Hospital, School of Nursing, in Kirksville, Missouri. Louise graduated in 1938 and Nelda graduated in 1944. Louise recalls some of her experiences in nursing school in the mid-1930s.

> I'm ninety years in November (2006). Tuition in school was $75 and this covered books and uniforms. I think that was the only fee ever but that was a goodly sum in 1935.

The nurses' home—only one bathroom in each home. We did it!! Nursing students occupied both of the nurses' homes.

Required age for entrance to the school of nursing was eighteen years of age. I applied in 1934 but lacked two months; therefore I entered in September 1935. Probation period was four months; we were called "probies." Uniforms were blue checked gingham with a white bib apron. No cap given until passed probation period and then the uniform was plain gray with white apron.

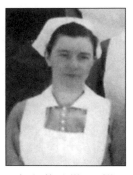

Louise Martin Warren, RN
[1938 *Osteoblast*, MOM]

We had classes four hours daily and floor duty four hours. Probies mopped each floor after patient trays were returned to the main kitchen on a manually operated dumb waiter. They had to soak bloody linens from the operating room in cold water in sitz bath tubs and wash the blood out before sending down to hospital laundry.

RE: Surgery, all linens were autoclaved. Surgical gloves and instruments were boiled and sharps immersed in alcohol. I do not recall ever having a post-operative infection.

We made our own cotton swabs and perineal pads, sharpened and re-used hypodermic needles, patched surgical gloves, and had a supply of rounded patches.

Anesthesia: Drip ether, usually given by the senior intern. Surgical team scrubbed to elbows and immersed in bichloride of mercury solution before gowns and gloves were put on. Patients usually remained in bed for ten days post-operatively; also OB patients remained in bed for ten days after delivery.

Our profession (DO) had wonderful results with pneumonia patients. The interns slept on the top floor of the hospital and got up each hour, day and night, and treated pneumonia patients osteopathically, thoracic area for fifteen minutes each hour. We cured <u>MANY</u> more patients than medical hospitals.[5]

Louise Martin Warren, RN, went on to work for many years as a nurse in several osteopathic hospitals. She recalls her first position as a surgical nurse at a "small, small" osteopathic hospital in Corpus Christi, Texas, in 1938. Her salary was $60 per month, plus room and board and laundering of uniforms. They worked twelve-hour shifts, with a half-day off each week and one day off each month. She was later joined in Corpus Christi by her sister Nelda and two class-mates.[6]

Nelda Martin Richardson, RN, recalls that during World War II there was an acute shortage of nurses and nursing students were frequently called upon to fill in for the lack of nurses in the hospital. She describes the need for bathing patients in bed since "early ambulation was not practiced." Nurses and student nurses were not allowed to take blood pressures or start IVs since this was reserved for externs, interns, or house physicians. Student nurses were required to mop patients' rooms and do most of the cleaning.

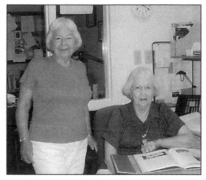

After graduation, Nelda continued to work at the Laughlin Hospital until she passed the state nursing boards. Nelda, along with two other newly licensed nurses, then went to Texas to join her sister at the Corpus Christi Osteopathic Hospital where they were short of surgical nurses. In September 1945, she moved to Portland, Maine, to marry Martyn Richardson, a 1945 graduate of the Kirksville

Seated: Louise Elaine (Martin) Warren, Laughlin Hospital School of Nursing class of 1938. Standing: Nelda M. (Martin) Richardson, Laughlin Hospital School of Nursing class of 1944. [author]

College of Osteopathy and Surgery who was serving his internship at the Osteopathic Hospital of Maine. Nelda notes that nine out of the fourteen members of her nursing school class married DOs.[7]

The Osteopathic Hospital of Philadelphia opened in 1911 and was affiliated with the Philadelphia College of Osteopathy. One of the purposes of the hospital was to run a training school for nurses. Lack of facilities delayed opening of the nursing school until 1915. With the opening of a larger hospital facility in 1917, the size of the class was increased from eight student nurses per class to twenty-one students. The nursing students did not pay tuition; instead they were trained in return for their services in the hospital. They worked nine hours a day and were given two weeks vacation. They did receive a small monthly allowance to help with their expenses. The entering students made their own uniforms, which consisted of a gingham blouse with a white skirt. They wore white shoes, stockings, and spats. The School of Nursing of the Osteopathic Hospital of Philadelphia was an

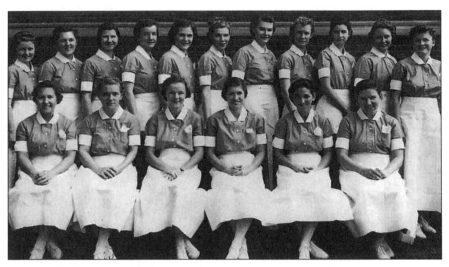

Osteopathic Hospital of Philadelphia, School of Nursing, class of 1942. [1996.156 PCOM]

integral part of the Philadelphia College of Osteopathy from 1915 until 1960. It was an officially recognized training school in the Commonwealth of Pennsylvania and upon graduation nurses were eligible for state board examination for the certificate of registered nurse.[8]

With the acquisition of the Woman's Homeopathic Hospital in 1951 and the existing 48th Street Hospital, Philadelphia College of Osteopathy reached a capacity of four hundred beds. The affiliation with Philadelphia General Hospital for medical, psychiatric, and pediatric training ensured that student nurses received ample clinical experience. Many osteopathic nurses served in military hospitals and medical facilities during World War II.[9] Due to financial reasons, the school of nursing closed in 1960. The educational program was one of the finest, as many of the instructors were members of the medical college faculty.

Among the last nursing students to graduate from the Philadelphia College of Osteopathy nursing school was Barbara Knosp. After graduation, Knosp

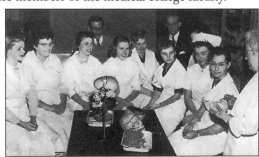

Second student from left is Barbara Knosp
[1957 *Osteopathic Digest*, PCOM]

moved to Lancaster, Pennsylvania, where she worked at the Lancaster Osteopathic Hospital (now known as Heart of Lancaster Medical Center) for her entire professional career, serving for many years as head nurse in the maternity department.[10]

Elizabeth Potter, RN

Not all nurses working in osteopathic hospitals were graduates of osteopathic training programs. Elizabeth Potter graduated from the St. Barnabas nursing program in 1937 and immediately took a position as a nurse at the Osteopathic Hospital of Maine where she worked until her retirement in 1978.

In 1954, while on leave to care for her ill father, Elizabeth responded to an urgent call by the hospital for nurses to care for an unusual delivery—the Pinkham quadruplets. For several weeks, Elizabeth assisted in providing round-the-clock private nursing care for the quadruplets. Her duties, in addition to nursing, were to inform the media of the babies' progress. Following the death of her father, Elizabeth returned to full-time nursing at the hospital. From 1957 until her retirement in 1978 she was the nursing supervisor for the 3 to 11 PM shift.

During the forty-one years that Nurse Potter was employed at the hospital, it grew from a 25-bed facility to a 136-bed hospital and was undergoing another expansion at the time of her retirement. From the time she began her career to when she retired, the hospital went from having a single intern to a flourishing internship program and residency programs in four specialties.[11]

NOTES

1. "The ASO," in *Osteoblast*, 1911, MOM; and Walter, *First School of Osteopathic Medicine*, 65.
2. "To Inspect the Mayo Hospital," *Journal of Osteopathy* 15, no. 10 (Oct. 1908): 638.
3. Walter, *First School of Osteopathic Medicine*, 102–3, 288.
4. Ibid., 102–3, 288.
5. Louise (Martin) Warren, "Memory Bits from Laughlin School of Nursing," personal correspondence with the author, ca. November 2006.
6. Ibid
7. Nelda (Martin) Richardson, personal correspondence with the author, 12 November 2006.
8. Perloff, *To Secure Merit*, 99–100.
9. Ibid, 100.
10. Barbara Knosp, RN, was a longtime professional associate and personal friend of the author.
11. Parker, *Historical Memoirs*, 24–27.

Chapter Nine
$\mathcal{W}$omen Influential to Osteopathic Medicine

"Of all the monikers that have been given to Dr. Still, *Liberator of Women* is the one I prefer."

Mary McClellan Burnett, DO

"No ignorant man or woman can get into our school, even though they roll in wealth."

Andrew Taylor Still, MD, DO

THROUGHOUT THE YEARS THERE HAVE BEEN NUMEROUS WOMEN who were not osteopathic physicians, but who have been beneficial, influential, or even indispensable to the osteopathic profession. Some were patients who were grateful for the benefits they received from osteopathic care that could not be obtained from orthodox medical care; some had other, unknown reasons for devoting themselves to the profession. Some supported the profession financially, some through their volunteer efforts, and some through their willingness to publicly support osteopathic medicine in its formative years. Some lent their expertise in other forms of medicine to the osteopathic profession, others used osteopathic techniques in their branch of medicine. It would be impossible to tell the stories of all of these women who have been important to osteopathic medicine; these are but a few of the women who deserve to be recognized.

EARLY SUPPORTERS OF DR. A. T. STILL
Family of A. T. Still
Growing up on the frontier, Andrew Taylor Still was surrounded by strong women. In the nineteenth century, women's lives were largely restricted to the domestic sphere, but for pioneer women like Martha Still, that domestic sphere included constant hard work. To make a comfortable home for their families in

primitive conditions, pioneer women cared for livestock, tended kitchen gardens and gathered food that grew wild, preserved food for the winter, sewed their family's clothing (often from cloth they had woven themselves), hauled water for cooking, cleaning, and washing, and made candles, soap, and other necessities. Andrew wrote that when his father was away on missionary trips, his mother "had to manage the farm, which she did as well as any one could. She spun, wove, cut and made clothing, butchered hogs or a beef, and managed it just as well as father, or a little better, for she was fully master of the situation." Frontier women were also responsible for teaching their children and creating a sense of civilization and culture in their community. In his autobiography, Still wrote of his mother, "She was my greatest friend while alive. She is the lighthouse of my chamber of reason."[1] Martha was a strong supporter of her son Andrew and his new science of osteopathy. She watched as he withdrew from the practice of allopathic medicine and developed his distinct form of medical practice. She witnessed Andrew's years of hardship; unfortunately, she did not live to see the opening of the first osteopathic medical school.[2]

Having witnessed the struggles of his frontier mother, the suffering and death of his first wife, and his second wife's heartache after the death of four children, Andrew knew firsthand the resilience of women in the face of hardship. Andrew's second wife, Mary Elvira Turner, was the daughter of a pharmacist and had assisted her father in the running of his small pharmacy, where she learned a good deal about sickness and compounding drugs. She often said that if women could have been doctors, she would surely have entered that profession. Mary Elvira first met Dr. A. T. Still when she was asked to examine a neighbor's sick children; she suspected they might have scarlet fever and advised the mother to call for a physician. She and Andrew married in November 1860.[3] In February 1865, three of Dr. Still's children from his first marriage died from meningitis, and Andrew and Mary Elvira's second child died of pneumonia (their first child had died in infancy). Dr. Still was devastated by the loss of his children, but together he and Mary Elvira began to rebuild their family and their lives. In 1865, they had a son, Charles; in 1867 twin sons, Herman and Harry; in 1874 a son, Fred; and in 1876 a daughter, Blanche.

Dr. Still's oldest child, Marusha, was the only child of his first marriage to survive to adulthood. When her brother and two sisters died of spinal meningitis, she was away from home visiting her grandparents. With her mother and siblings dead, Marusha did not return home and was the only child of Andrew Still who did not study to become an osteopathic physician. However, she married and her two sons received their DO degrees at the American School of Osteopathy.

As Andrew gradually withdrew from the practice of allopathic medicine and started to explore therapeutic alternatives, he was shunned by his fellow physicians. Even his brothers, who were allopathic physicians, rejected his new form of treatment. Patients feared the unfamiliar and unproven methods he was using, and Baker University, which the Still family had helped to build, rejected his request to teach his new science. In church, the presiding elder, a former president of Baker University, denounced Still and his theories, describing him as an "apostate of the first water" who must either "change his tactics or land in hell."[4] Through all of these troubles, Mary Elvira stood by his side.

After relocating to Kirksville, when Andrew was not able to support his family, Mary Elvira sold magazine subscriptions and the boys found odd jobs when they could. Poverty became a way of life, and soon Andrew was forced to become a migrant physician, traveling from town to town promoting his new science of osteopathy and trying to earn enough money to support his family. Finally, Dr. Still began to be accepted in the community, but tragedy struck again when he developed a severe case of typhoid fever. For months he was bedridden and unable to practice. Mary Elvira nursed him, and she and the children again took on additional work to support the family, this time with the help of local townspeople who had benefited from his treatments.[5] This was a trying period for Mary Elvira, and it was her strength and fortitude that held the family together during Dr. Still's incapacitation.

Mary Elvira never lost faith in her husband's ambitions. She witnessed the opening of the first osteopathic medical college, with all of their five children as members of that first class of the American School of Osteopathy. She was an active part of the early osteopathic profession; early classes of osteopathic students affectionately called her "Mother Osteopathy." As their financial fortunes changed, Andrew built Mary Elvira a large home on Osteopathy Street directly across from the college, where they lived until her death in 1910.

Julia Ivie

In the 1870s, Julia Ivie owned a small hotel on the north side of the town square in Kirksville, Missouri. In March 1875, a traveling physician by the name of Andrew Taylor Still, commonly known as the "tramp doctor,"[6] arrived in the small northeast Missouri town with no money, no practice, no office, and no place to live. Julia Ivie gave Dr. Still free room and board at the Ivie Hotel[7] for a month to help him get started. In his autobiography, Dr. Still affectionately refers to her as Mother Ivie.[8] But Julia Ivie was not alone in her efforts. Charlie Chinn donated office space where Dr. Still could start treating patients. Dr. F. A. Grove, Judge Linder, and Mr. Robert Harris also gave assistance and support until Dr. Still could establish a practice and send for his family to join him.

Mrs. J. K. Mitchell

Another supporter in the early 1870s was Mrs. J. K. Mitchell, wife of a Presbyterian minister in Kirksville. After a fall from a horse, her young daughter had lost the ability to walk. The concerned parents had taken her to multiple physicians who examined her and tried everything they knew, but nothing worked. With orthodox physicians unable to help the child, Mrs. Mitchell implored her husband to allow her to take the child to the new practitioner in town, but her husband refused. He had heard stories about this new doctor who dressed in baggy, disheveled clothing and walked around with a bag of human bones that he would pull out to demonstrate how he adjusted bones to make people better. No respectable person in town would be treated by him. No matter how much Mrs. Mitchell pleaded, the minister refused to allow her to take their daughter to see Dr. Still.

When her husband was out of town, a desperate Mrs. Mitchell took her daughter to see Dr. Still. After examining the child, Dr. Still determined that the problem was a dislocated hip. He manipulated the girl's spine and pelvis and immediately, after the hip was replaced, the child was able to walk. When Rev. Mitchell returned home, he was amazed to see that his daughter was walking normally. That Sunday Rev. Mitchell took his daughter to church and from the pulpit showed his parishioners how the child was now able to walk normally. The minister explained that Dr. A. T. Still had treated the child and restored her ability to walk. Dr. Still's practice immediately improved and soon he no longer had to travel to other towns to find patients.[9]

Helen de Lendrecie

The testimonies of grateful patients did much to support the new profession of osteopathic medicine. Helen de Lendrecie lived in Fargo, North Dakota, where she became involved in the fight for the right of osteopaths to be licensed in that state. She told her story in an 1897 letter to the *Journal of Osteopathy*.

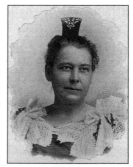

Helen de Lendrecie
[1897 *Journal of Osteopathy*, MOM]

> In the fall of 1895 a lump appeared in my right breast. Our family physician advised its immediate removal assuring me that nothing but the knife could remedy

the evil and stating that it would soon assume a malignant form if not removed without delay. Knowing him to be a fine surgeon as well as a physician, I placed myself in his hands and submitted to an operation whereby my entire breast was removed. It was a great shock to my nervous system, and I had not recovered from it, when the same trouble appeared in my left breast. I had heard meantime of osteopathy and resolved to try it before again submitting to the knife.... I went to Kirksville and was completely cured in six weeks time. My own eyes saw and my own hand felt the obstruction that caused the trouble in both cases, and I knew very well that the knife was never necessary.... Osteopathy has clearly proven its right to recognition in the healing of cases heretofore declared only curable by the knife, and it is only right that its supporters should sustain its claim.[10]

Helen de Lendrecie spoke before the North Dakota State Senate when the osteopathic licensing bill came up for a vote. In spite of arguments against the bill by the MDs, the North Dakota Senate passed the bill. The governor, also an osteopathic patient, signed the licensing bill into law.

Helen de Lendrecie had no medical training and explained her medical condition in nonmedical terms, so it is difficult to know exactly what her pathology was or how it was cured using osteopathic manipulation. The only hints we have are that the lump was initially found in her right breast, and she later developed a similar lump in her left breast. She stated that the lumps were caused by an "obstruction," possibly a word she heard used by Helen Peterson, DO, who treated her at the osteopathic infirmary in Kirksville.[11] Whatever the cause of the "obstruction," it is obvious that surgery was not necessary and the condition could be alleviated by noninvasive osteopathic treatments. An educated guess would be that it was a blockage of the lymphatic ducts or venous blood drainage, but we can never know for sure.

Julia Foraker

In 1895, the American School of Osteopathy and the infirmary in Kirksville had earned a reputation in the three-state area of Missouri, Iowa, and Illinois, but was mostly unknown outside of that region, that is until US Senator and Mrs. Joseph P. Foraker of Ohio brought their son, Arthur, to Kirksville seeking treatment. After a few months, the boy, who had been treated without results

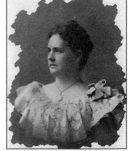

Julia Foraker
[1897 *Journal of Osteopathy*, MOM]

at leading medical centers throughout the country, began to show improvement. Mrs. Julia Foraker was so pleased with the results that she purchased a home in Kirksville and lived there for three years while her son was under osteopathic treatment. In 1897, she told a reporter:

> My opinion of Osteopathy has been published in a former issue of the *Journal*, and I have no reason to change it. Arthur continues to improve, and we feel very hopeful of a complete cure. In addition to the benefits received in my own family, I have witnessed many wonderful cures during my stay in Kirksville. This new practice is not a fad but a science well worthy of the attention of the scientific world. I am a friend of Osteopathy and shall do all in my power to promote its success everywhere.[12]

When her friend Col. A. L. Conger, chairman of the Republican National Committee, had a stroke, Mrs. Foraker convinced him to come to Kirksville and be treated osteopathically. Mrs. Conger was so impressed with the improvement in her husband's condition that she became an osteopathic physician (see p. 63).

During the three years she lived in Kirksville, Mrs. Foraker helped organize social activities for local women and female patients temporarily residing in Kirksville while receiving treatment at the osteopathic infirmary. In 1897, she founded the Sojourners Club, which is still active in local service activities. The Sojourners Club used the Osteopathic Infirmary building to house their private library and meeting rooms for visitors to interact with locals residents. Other charter members of the Sojourners Club were Anna Still, Blanche Still, and the wife of Judge Ellison.

Mae Critchfield

Another satisfied patient allowed her history to be reported in the November 1898 issue of the *Journal of Osteopathy*.

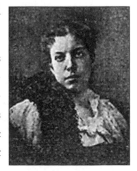

> The young lady whose portrait accompanies this sketch is a living illustration of the virtue of perseverance. Her recent visit to this city where she is so popular and where she has formed so many friendships among our young society people has renewed public interest in her remarkable cure through osteopathy at the A. T. Still Infirmary.
>
> Miss Mae Critchfield, of Oskaloosa, Kansas, came to the infirmary on the 17th of April, 1895. Her

Mae Critchfield
[November 1898 *Journal of Osteopathy*, MOM]

home physician advised against her coming, because her condition was such that they did not believe that she could survive the fatigue of the journey. In the preceding February she had a severe attack of cerebro-spinal meningitis, lying unconscious for fourteen days. The disease left her in a pitiable condition. One hip was dislocated and the upper left portion of the body was paralyzed from the center of the back. She could not lift her left arm, and one side of her neck being paralyzed, it was necessary that her head should be propped up when not in a recumbent position. She was unable to sit up but a small part of the time, and the left part of her body was totally insensible, so that even pin pricks were not felt. It was in this condition that osteopathy found Miss Critchfield. Today, no more sprightly, active and happy young lady can be met with in many a day's journey. But much of the credit of this wonderful transformation must be given to Miss. Critchfield herself. Through the long months of preparatory treatment, thirty-two, we believe—her perseverance and faith did not waiver. There was a constant and steady, though apparently slow improvement. The muscles were drawn and contracted and it took a long time to restore them to their normal condition. From July to November 1897 she went upon crutches, but at last her patience and perseverance were to be fully rewarded. The Saturday mail of November 13th, 1897, gives the climax of the case as follows:

On last Monday something startling occurred. It was so startling that it even scared Dr. Harry Still, the operator, and all in the operating room. We don't know anything about osteopathic or anatomic terms. We only know from our interview with Miss Mae, that the hip was set; the proper bones were put in place, and she walks today with only the slight-est trace of a limp. A happier girl it would be hard to find. As her mother says, "It is hard to realize that what we have been hoping and praying for has come to pass. You can hardly imagine our gratitude."

During Miss. Critchfield's recent visit to Kirksville, she was a fre-quent visitor to the infirmary. In an interview with the writer, she kindly consented to the publication of her portrait and a recapitulation of her case. She declares that she is perfectly restored to health and activity, and that she has experienced no return of her trouble since she left for her home in Kansas some months ago. It is hardly necessary to add that osteopathy has no warmer or more enthusiastic advocate than Miss Mae Critchfield, of Oskaloosa, Kansas. At her own request we add in conclu-sion that she desires proper credit to be given Drs. A. T. Still, Harry Still, and Dr. Landes, now of Michigan, for the first months of her treatment, and to Dr. Harry Still and Dr. Gentry for the completion of her cure.[13]

Phoebe T. Williamson, MD

The Philadelphia College and Infirmary of Osteopathy was opened in January 1899 by Mason Presley, DO, who initially taught all the classes himself. He was joined in May 1899 by O. J. Snyder, DO, who then shared the teaching. By January 1900, the faculty expanded to eight professors, including four MDs, one of whom was Phoebe Williamson, MD. There were relatively few female MDs at the end of the nineteenth century, let alone a female MD teaching at an osteopathic medical school. Dr. Williamson, a graduate of the Woman's Medical College of New York Infirmary, was the first female faculty member at the Philadelphia College and Infirmary of Osteopathy. She lectured on obstetrics and gynecology.

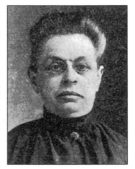

Phoebe T. Williamson, MD
[1900 *Philadelphia Journal of Osteopathy*, PCOM]

With a relatively low student enrollment in the early years, income from tuition and fees could not pay salaries for professors and instructors. Instead of receiving cash, the faculty accepted shares of Philadelphia College and Infirmary of Osteopathy stock; one share for thirty-three hours of instruction. The addition of the extra faculty added more specialized teaching and allowed Drs. Presley and Snyder to develop a clinical practice in the school infirmary, which brought additional revenue and provided a diversity of clinical experience for the medical students.[14]

Grace Noll Crowell

In 1938, Grace Noll Crowell wrote a poem dedicated to the osteopathic physicians of America, which she read at the American Osteopathic Association annual convention in Dallas, Texas. Crowell was a well-known and popular poet who published thirty-six books of poetry and whose works appeared in hundreds of newspapers and magazines. In 1935, she was named poet laureate of Texas, a position she held for three years. In 1938, she was awarded the Golden Scroll Medal of Honor as National Honor Poet, the Golden Rule Foundation selected her as American Mother of the Year, and *American Women*, a biographical publication, selected her as one of ten Outstanding American Women. While her connection to osteopathic medicine is not known, she wrote that she had suffered from "a long series of ill-nesses" after the birth of her first child and had visited numerous doctors looking for relief. It is tempting to speculate that she was inspired by stories of successful treatments by osteopathic physicians when she wrote this poem.[15]

Hands

You give your strong and vital hands to find the source of pain;
your touch is quick and sure, and as delicate as the fingers of the blind,
as you explore dark lanes and seek to cure the ancient secret pains that torture
    men,
the old, old agonies that stalk the lands, you wrestle with them all,
and once again hurt bodies straighten, healed beneath your hands.

Your hearts and minds are kindled with a flame:
A zeal to win where others fail.
You know the body's desperate need; you have a name you would uphold;
in numbers you would grow until, new visioned, all the world may see
and seek the help of Osteopathy.

CELEBRITY SUPPORTERS OF OSTEOPATHY

As any good advertiser will tell you, support from prominent people goes far in promoting a product or service. For the young science of osteopathy, public state-ments of support were important, and were often noted in professional journals. In February 1939, the *Journal of Osteopathy* reported that writer Somerset Maugham had arrived in the United States and "explained to newspapermen upon his arrival in New York that he had been lured to this country by the fame of New York Osteopaths." Maugham had been injured in a automobile accident and "wanted Osteopathic care."[16]

In August 1939, the *Forum of Osteopathy* reported that movie star Greer Gar-son "likes osteopathy." The actress had been sick and reported that doctors "said I had something wrong with my spine." She saw an osteopathic physician, "who fixed my spine. I made the picture and I've felt fine ever since." Later that year, the journal reported that Helen B. Jones, DO, was in charge of the Emergency Hospital at MGM studios in California, noting that the chief surgeon at the downtown hospi-tal where MGM employees were insured had "expressed complete satisfaction with the service that is being rendered."[17]

In May 1948, at the height of her career, Academy Award–winning actress Bette Davis gave birth to her daughter in the Santa Anna Community Hospital, which was an osteopathic institution. The physician who delivered her child was Vincent P. Carroll, DO (Kirksville College of Osteopathy and Surgery, 1919). The actress was so pleased with the care she and her daughter had received at the hospital that she made a donation to the hospital building fund of $10,000, a sizable amount in 1948.[18]

Osteopathy has had numerous supporters among the British royal family as well. In 1940, the *Forum of Osteopathy* noted a report by CBS foreign correspondent Ed Murrow that Queen Elizabeth, while visiting Birmingham, suffered from a stiff neck. She "was treated by an American osteopath, and feels much better." The article also noted a wire story reporting the same events and adding that the doctor who treated the queen was Dr. Elmer T. Pheils, a 1905 graduate of the American School of Osteopathy and former president of the British Osteopathic Association.[19]

Royal support for osteopathy in Britain has continued into the twenty-first century. Diana Frances Spencer, who was married to Charles, Prince of Wales, was respected worldwide for her tireless efforts for charity and for her warmth and humanity. In her multiple charitable endeavors, one theme was repeated time and time again—her deep love of children. Following her untimely death, the Diana Princess of Wales Fund granted London's Osteopathic Centre for Children the sum of one million pounds. This generous endowment was in recognition that Diana had been scheduled to launch the charity's Sweet Pea Appeal to raise money for a new facility in London, which took place just days after her death. The Osteopathic Centre for Children, London was established in 1991 and at the time of Diana's involvement with the center, was treating twenty-five thousand pediatric patients a year. It is the only center for pediatric osteopathy in Europe. Diana had served as the president of the General Council and Register of Osteopaths, and Prince Charles served as the president of the General Osteopathic Council.[20]

Princess Anne, the only daughter of Queen Elizabeth II of England, has frequently been referred to as the hardest working member of the House of Windsor. She is an athlete and an accomplished equestrian, winning several titles and medals and representing Great Britain in the Montreal Olympics. Princess Anne is also an ardent and active supporter of osteopathy. Since 1984, she has been the Royal Patron of the British School of Osteopathy, the oldest osteopathic college in Great Britain, and participates in many of the school's events, including presenting diplomas to graduates.

In 2005, the British School of Osteopathy formed an exclusive partnership with the University of Luton that enabled osteopathic students to pay standard fees rather than private costs, saving them thousands of pounds every year for their osteopathic education. At the November graduation, Princess Anne awarded degrees to over one hundred graduates. In her remarks to the graduates, Princess Anne stated, "The reputation and understanding of osteopathy will come via those who pass through the school. Osteopathy is a very important part of healthcare in this country." She expressed interest in "seeing how public funding would widen participation and encourage even more students from a range of backgrounds to enter the profession." In November 2010, the Princess Royal presented the first-ever Master of Osteopathy degrees to graduates of the British School of Osteopathy and University of Bedfordshire. [21]

OSTEOPATHIC HISTORIAN
Georgia Warner Walter

Few people have ever been awarded honorary DO degrees, and probably the only husband and wife team ever to receive this honor are Georgia Walter and her husband, Bucky Walter. Georgia W. Walter's father, Maxwell Warner, graduated from the A. T. Still College of Osteopathy and Surgery in 1925. He decided to become an osteopath after he was treated by osteopathic physicians who restored his ability to walk after he suffered atrophy of his left leg and right arm as a result of influenza during the pandemic of 1918/19. Dr. Warner taught at the Kirksville College of Osteopathy and Surgery and in 1940 became the dean of the college, a position he held for seventeen years.

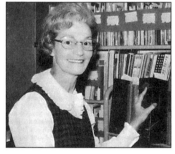

Georgia W. Walter, director of the A. T. Still Library 1969–1986
[A. T. Still University]

Georgia had attended Northeast Missouri State Teachers College in Kirksville (now Truman State University) and later obtained her librarian certificate. She married Francis "Bucky" Walter, who was with the Kirksville College of Osteopathic Medicine for thirty-five years. Georgia was the librarian at the Kirksville College of Osteopathic Medicine from 1969 until she retired in 1986. In that year, Georgia and her husband were awarded honorary doctor of osteopathic education degrees by the Kirksville College of Osteopathic Medicine.

Georgia served on the American Osteopathic Association College Accrediting Team for five years. In 1987, the Kirksville College of Osteopathic Medicine awarded her the Living Tribute Award and named the library reading room in her honor. In November 2005, the Missouri Humanities Council awarded her the Governor's Book Award for *The First School of Osteopathic Medicine*. Georgia published many articles and gave lectures on the history of osteopathic medicine; in addition to her book, she published several booklets: "The First D.O.," "Women in Osteopathic Medicine," and "Osteopathic Medicine Past and Present."[22]

ANIMAL OSTEOPATHS

Lu Ann Groves, DVM

A. T. Still probably never envisioned osteopathic techniques being used on horses, but there is no reason the same principles that work so well for humans should not be used for the treatment of animals. Veterinarian Dr. Lu Ann Groves runs the Whole Horse Texas Center for Equine Care and Education at the Whole Horse Veterinary Clinic in San Marcos. After receiving her doctorate in veterinary medicine, Dr. Groves graduated from the W2E2 School for Equine Osteopathy conducted by Janek

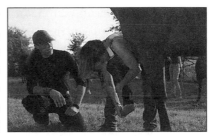

Veterinarian Dr. Lu Ann Groves performing osteopathic manipulative therapy on a horse, under the direction of Janek Vluggen, DO.

Vluggen, DO. Dr. Vluggen received his DO degree from the International Academy of Osteopathy, Gent, Belgium.[23]

Dr. Groves uses osteopathy to look at the whole horse in terms of endocrine and immune function, and to ensure balance in the autonomic nervous system. Osteopathy can help caregivers prevent sickness by recognizing early signs of disharmony in the horse, and to increase the level of performance and well-being of healthy animals. In some cases, an osteopathic treatment can correct lameness, or clear blockages in tissues or organs.

Emily Bewsey

Emily Bewsey has always had a keen interest in animals, especially horses. She has worked with horses in England, America, and Australia for many years. In 2005, she graduated with a first class honors degree in osteopathy and went on to complete the postgraduate course in animal osteopathy at the Osteopathic Centre for Animals conducted by Stuart McGregor, one of the world's leading equine osteopaths. In total, it took her six years of training to qualify as an animal osteopath.

Emily feels that osteopathy provides a holistic approach that enables her to treat humans and animals successfully.

The osteopathic treatment of horses has many similarities to the treatment of humans. The initial consultation begins by creating a case history, noting any previous injuries, treatments, and medications, as well as looking at the lifestyle of the horse and the demands placed on it. The equine osteopath then observes the horse in-hand, at walk, and trot, and asks it to perform a series of turns. Depending on the problem, the osteopath may require the horse to be lunged and/or ridden. She then conducts an osteopathic examination of the horse, assessing the joints, including the spine, muscles, ligaments, and tendons. After a careful history and physical examination, and consultation with the horse's owner and veterinarian, the animal osteopath provides appropriate treatment.

Dr. Bewsey is not the only equine osteopath in the United Kingdom, nor is she the only female equine osteopath. The International Association of Equine Osteopaths lists equine osteopaths in the UK, Australia, Canada, Europe, Israel, and the United States. The organization has a certification program to ensure that practitioners meet standards of practice and competency in areas including parietal, visceral, and cranialsacral techniques. Dr. Bewsey is registered with the General Osteopathic Council and is a member of the British Osteopathic Association. In addition to her practice as an animal osteopath, she also conducts a purely human osteopathic practice. [24]

NOTES

1. Still, *Autobiography*, 454–56.
2. Trowbridge, *Andrew Taylor Still*, 7–8, 11, 27, 43–44.
3. Ibid., 85–86, 92, 200–201; and C. E. Still, *Frontier Doctor, Medical Pioneer*, 80–83.
4. Still, "Recollections of Baldwin, Kansas," *Journal of Osteopathy* 1, no. 9 (Jan. 1895): 2; and Trowbridge, *Andrew Taylor Still*, 125–38.
5. C. E. Still, *Frontier Doctor, Medical Pioneer*, 95–98, 103, 105.
6. Violette, *History of Adair County*, 248.
7. March, *Book of Adair County History*, 322.
8. Still, *Autobiography*, 124–25.
9. C. E. Still, *Frontier Doctor, Medical Pioneer*, 101; Bunting, "How Osteopathy Got Its First Recognition in Kirksville," *Journal of Osteopathy* 5, no. 10 (March 1899): 473–75; and Hildreth, *Lengthening Shadow of Dr. Andrew Taylor Still*, 13–15.
10. "A Brilliant Legislative Victory," *Journal of Osteopathy* 4 (June 1897): 81–83.
11. Alice Patterson-Shelby, DO, Collection, MOM.
12. "Some Osteopathic Results," *Journal of Osteopathy* 4, no. 2 (June–Dec. 1897): 289.
13. "Perseverence Rewarded," *Journal of Osteopathy* 5, no. 6 (Nov. 1898): 273–74.
14. Perloff, *To Secure Merit*, 3–4.
15. "Grace Noll Crowell: Songs out of Suffering," 181.

16. "Sullivan and Maugham," *Journal of Osteopathy* 46 (Feb. 1939); 8.

17. "Garson Was a Goner," *Forum of Osteopathy* 13 (Aug. 1939): 98; and "Current News: D. O. Heads M-G-M Emergency Hospital," *Forum of Osteopathy* 13 (Sept. 1939): 131–32.

18. Walter, *First School of Osteopathic Medicine*, 280.

19. "In the Mailbag: Royalty's Neck," *Forum of Osteopathy* 14 (June 1940): 50.

20. BBC News, "Diana Fund Announces Grants," 10 March 1998, accessed 17 March 2007, http://news.bbc.co.uk/2/hi/uk_news/63743.stm; and Bala Health Clinic, "Training, Registration, and Status," accessed 3 Nov. 2006, www.balahealth.com/.

21. "Official Website of the British Monarchy, The Princess Royal," accessed 5 Jan. 2011, www.royal.gov.uk/ThecurrentRoyalFamily/ThePrincessRoyal/ThePrincessRoyal. aspx. See also University of Bedfordshire, "Princess Royal Presents Degrees to First Osteopathy Graduates," 24 November 2005, accessed 17 March 2007, www.beds.ac.uk/news/2005/nov/051124-bso; and University of Bedfordshire, "Royal Seal of Approval for Uni Graduates," 11 November 2010, accessed 5 Jan. 2011, www.beds.ac.uk/news/2010/nov/101111-bso.

22. Georgia W. Walter, personal interview with the author, 17 September 2006.

23. Lu Ann Groves, DVM, personal correspondence with the author, 8 June 2007.

24. Emily O'Sullivan (Bewsey), personal correspondence with the author, 29 January 2007; and Bewsey, "Equine Osteopathy," accessed 5 Feb. 2007, www.equine-osteopathy. org.uk/page4.html.

Glossary

allopathy/allopathic medicine: a system of medicine in which a disease is treated by using remedies (such as drugs or surgery) that produce effects that are different or incompatible with the condition being treated. The term *allopathic medicine* was coined by Samuel Hahnemann in 1810 to differentiate conventional medicine from *homeopathic medicine*, since both types of physicians used the MD degree. The term was used primarily by physicians with unconventional training as a pejorative term for conventional practitioners. The term is also used by osteopathic physicians to refer to practitioners with an MD degree, but practitioners with an MD degree do not commonly use the term to describe themselves.

bloody flux: archaic term for dysentery, a form of bloody diarrhea.

bonesetting: a form of treatment popular in the early nineteenth century that focused on treating dislocations and fractures. Practitioners were called *bonesetters*. Because the procedures could be painful, many practitioners called themselves *lightening bonesetters* to indicate that they were lightening fast, so the patient would experience less pain.

chiropractic: a system of therapy based on the idea that disease results from a lack of normal nerve function, and employs manipulation and adjustment to restore normal function.

cranial therapy / craniosacral therapy / cranial sacral therapy: A form of manipulation of the head and spine developed by William Sutherland, DO. Used for infants and children before the fusing of the cranial bones. The effectiveness of this therapy in adults remains controversial.

DOCARE: An osteopathic medical outreach program providing healthcare to indigent and isolated people around the world.[1] Full name is DOCARE International.

eclecticism/eclectic medicine: a branch of American medicine that grew out of Thomsonian medicine in the early nineteenth century, and used indigenous plants and botanical remedies, along with physical therapy to treat the symptoms of a disease. The term was coined by Constantine Samuel Rafinesque—a physician who observed Native Americans' use of medicinal plants—to describe physicians who used whatever methods were found to benefit their patients, but opposed heroic methods such as bleeding, purging, and the use of mercury compounds.

electronic medicine: a form of medical practice based on the theories of Albert Abrams, MD, who theorized that every disease has a specific vibration that can be measured and treated by duplication of the electronic vibration, thus neutralizing the disease. What he called the Electronic Reactions of Abrams (ERA) used an "Oscilloclast"(meaning "vibration breaker"), also called an Abrams Machine, to diagnose and treat patients using electrodes. Abrams's theories were challenged by both osteopathic and medical physicians, and proven to be ineffective. The ERA scam is widely considered one of the greatest medical hoaxs of all time.[2]

heroic medicine: extraordinary measures taken to treat a patient, that included bleeding the patient to the point of unconsciousness, purging, and the use of mercury and arsenic compounds.

homeopathy/homeopathic medicine: a therapeutic system developed by Samuel Hahnemann in Germany in the early nineteenth century, based on the "law of similars" (like cures like), which holds that medical substances will evoke certain symptoms in a healthy person that will heal an illness having similar symptoms as the medication administered. Homeopathy also applies the "law of infinitesimals" (the more the medication is diluted the more powerful the result).[3]

lymphatic pump: an osteopathic manipulative technique designed to increase the flow of lymphatic fluid. Recent research has revealed that this technique increases the number of leukocytes in the circulating lymphatic fluid and blood.[4]

magnetic healer: archaic term for a person who heals with their hands.

materia medica: the origin and preparation of medications.[5] Referring to medication and/or any therapeutic agents.

nosocomial: a condition associated with being in a hospital.

osteopath: "A person who has achieved the nationally-recognized academic and professional standards within her or his country to independently practice, diagnose, and provide treatment based upon the principles of osteopathic philosophy."[6]

osteopathic manipulative therapy (OMT): "The therapeutic application of manually guided forces by an osteopathic physician to improve the physiological function and/or support homeostasis that have been altered by somatic dysfunction."[7]

osteopathy/osteopathic medicine: "A complete system of medical care with a philosophy that combines the needs of the patient with the current practice of medicine, surgery, and obstetrics; that emphasizes the interrelationship between structure and function; and has an appreciation of the body's ability to heal itself."[8]

phrenology: a theory developed by German physician Franz Joseph Gall in 1796 that different parts of the brain are associated with specific mental faculties, and that the shape of the skull conforms to the size and shape of these parts, and that a phrenologist could determine an individual's personality traits, character, and propensities by measuring the area of the skull that overlies the corresponding area of the brain. Phrenology was especially popular in the early nineteenth century, but by the late nineteenth century, was widely considered a pseudoscience.

physiomedical: a form of botanical medicine that grew out of Thomsonian medicine.[9]

regular physicians/regulars: a term used by so-called *allopathic physicians* to distinguish themselves from so-called *irregular physicians* such as *homeopathic*, *eclectic*, and *osteopathic physicians*.[10]

somatic: Related to or involving the bones, muscles, nerves, and connective tissue of the body.[11]

somatic dysfunction: "Impaired or altered function of related components of the somatic system"[12]

Thomsonianism/Thomsonian medicine: a medical reform movement founded by Samuel Thomson in the early 1800s. The Thomsonian System was based on the use of herbal remedies and treatments such as steambaths and purging to remove toxins from the body. Thomson used only plants that grew towards the sun and signified heat, light and life, and rejected minerals because they came from the earth and signified illness and death.[13] As part of the popular health movement, the Thomsonian movement did not believe in formal education for physicians, but held that anyone could use the Thomsonian System to treat themselves and their family. Physiomedical and eclectic medicine were outgrowths of Thomsonianism.

NOTES

1. DOCARE, accessed 21 July 2009, http://www.docareintl.org/home/html.

2. See Armstrong and Armstrong, *Great American Medicine Show*, 193.

3. Spraycar, *Stedman's Medical Dictionary*, 26th ed., 804; and Armstrong and Armstrong, *Great American Medicine Show*, 33.

4. DiGiovanna and Schiowitz, *Encyclopedia of Osteopathy*, 61; and Hodge et al., "Lymphatic Pump Treatment Increases Leukocyte Numbers in Thoracic Duct Lymph," *JAOA* 106, no. 8 (Aug. 2006): 496.

5. Spraycar, *Stedman's Medical Dictionary*, 26th edition., 1069

6. World Osteopathic Health Organization, accessed 2 July 2009, http://www.woho.org/.

7. Ward, *Foundations for Osteopathic Medicine*, 1240.

8. Definition of osteopathic medicine, as reaffirmed by the American Osteopathic Association House of Delegates, 2003.

9. Armstrong and Armstrong, *Great American Medicine Show*, 258.

10. Booth, *History of Osteopathy*, 242.

11. Spraycar, *Stedman's Medical Dictionary*, 26th ed., 1634.

12. Ward, *Foundations for Osteopathic Medicine*, 1249.

13. Armstrong and Armstrong, *Great American Medicine Show*, 11.

Works Cited

"A. T. Still Infirmary." *Journal of Osteopathy* 4 (June 1897): frontispiece.

Abrams, Albert. *New Concepts in Diagnosis and Treatment*. San Francisco: Self, 1916.

"ACOS Inaugurates New President during Annual Conference Ceremonial Conclave." *ACOS News* 44 (Oct. 2006): 1–5.

Adler, Philip, and George W. Northup, eds. *100 Years of Osteopathic Medicine*. Northfield, IL: Medical Communications, 1978.

Allison, J. S. "My Impression of the Flu." *Journal of Osteopathy* 26 (July 1919): 289–91.

American Association of Colleges of Osteopathic Medicine. *2006 Annual Statistical Report on Osteopathic Medical Education*. Chevy Chase, MD: American Association of Colleges of Osteopathic Medicine, 2006.

American Chiropractic Association. "What is Chiropractic?" Accessed 7 July 2010, www.acatoday.org/level2_ccs.cfm?T1D=13&T2ED=61.

American National Biography. 24 vols. Edited by John A. Garraty and Mark C. Carnes. New York: Oxford University Press, 1999.

American Osteopathic Association. *AOA Daily Report*, 21 April 2009 and 19 July 2009.

———. *AOA Fact Sheet* for 1965, 1967, 1991, and 2006.

———. *AOA Yearbook and Directory of Osteopathic Physicians* for 1913, 1923, and 1979–80.

———. "Historic Reference of Osteopathic Colleges." Accessed 18 Feb. 2011. history.osteopathic.org/collegehist.shtml.

———. *The History of Osteopathic Medicine Virtual Museum*. Accessed 17 Feb. 2011. history.osteopathic.org/.

———. *The People and Events that Shaped Our History: A Centennial Perspective, 1897–1997*. Chicago: AOA, 1997.

———. "Years States Passed Unlimited Practice Laws." *AOA, History of Osteopathic Medicine Virtual Museum*. Accessed 30 Jan. 2009. history.osteopathic.org/laws.shtml.

"American Osteopathic Relief Association." *Journal of Osteopathy* 24 (May 1917): 278–84.

Anderson, Gunnar, et al., "A Comparison of Osteopathic Spinal Manipulation with Standard Care for Patients with Low Back Pain." *New England Journal of Medicine* 341, no. 19 (Nov. 1999): 1426–31.

"AOA Charters New Group." *AOA News Bulletin* 4 (Feb. 1961): 1.

Appointment of Doctors of Osteopathy as Medical Officers. Hearings on HR 483 Before a Subcommitee of the Committee on Armed Services. US Senate, 84th Cong., 2nd sess. Washington DC: Government Printing Office, 1956.

Armenta, Kin. "Unit 2: Osteopathic Medicine's Experiment at Los Angeles County General Hospital." *The DO* 50, no. 5 (2009): 44.

Armstrong, David, and Elizabeth Metzger Armstrong. *The Great American Medicine Show: Being an Illustrated History of Hucksters, Healers, Health Evangelists, and Heroes from Plymouth Rock to the Present*. New York: Prentice Hall, 1991.

"Asks if A. T. Still Ever Was a Real Doctor." *Osteopathic Physician* 15 (1909): 8.

"ASO to Adopt Three Year Course." *Journal of Osteopathy* 12 (Jan. 1905): 1.

Baker, Helen. "Female Enrollment in Colleges of Osteopathic Medicine: Five Years and Five Percentage Points Behind." *JAOA* 95 (Oct. 1995): 604–6.

Bala Health Clinic. "Training, Registration, and Status." Accessed 3 Nov. 2006. www.bala-health.com/.

Barge, James H., et al., "Osteopathy: Special Report of the Judicial Council to the AMA House of Delegates." *JAMA* 177 (1961): 774–76.

Bartosh, Louisa. "The History of Osteopathy in California." *Journal of the Osteopathic Physicians and Surgeons of California* 5 (April–May 1978): 30–33.

BBC News. "Diana Fund Announces Grants," 10 March 1998. Accessed 17 March 2007. http://news.bbc.co.uk/2/hi/uk_news/63743.stm.

Beal, Myron C. "Foreword." *American Academy of Osteopathy Yearbook* (1994): iv.

"Beginning of the Research Movement." *Osteopathic Physician* 14 (Dec. 1908): 11–12.

Bewsey, Emily (O'Sullivan). "Equine Osteopathy." Accessed 5 Feb. 2007. www.equine-osteopathy.org.uk/page4.html.

Bolles, Jeanette Hubbard. "Dr. Still's Regard for Woman's Ability." *JAOA* 17 (Jan. 1918): 250.

Bonner, Thomas Neville. *To the Ends of the Earth: Women's Search for Education in Medicine.* Cambridge, MA: Harvard University Press, 1992.

"Book Reviews." *Journal of Osteopathy* 23 (Jan. 1916): 58.

Booker, Anton S. *Wildcats in Petticoats: A Garland of Female Desperadoes—Lizzie Merton, Zoe Wilkins, Flora Quick Mundis, Bonnie Parker, Katie Bender and Belle Starr,* 8–10. Girard, KS: Haldeman-Julius Publications, 1945.

Booth, Emmons Rutledge. *History of Osteopathy and Twentieth-Century Medical Practice.* Cincinnati, OH: Caxton Press, 1905.

"A Brilliant Legislative Victory." *Journal of Osteopathy* 4, no. 2 (June 1897): 81–83.

Bunting, Henry S. "How Osteopathy Got Its First Recognition in Kirksville." *Journal of Osteopathy* 5 (March 1899): 473–75.

———, ed. "Science Offers New Field for the Blind." *Journal of Osteopathy* 5 (March 1899): 490.

Burbick, Joan. *Healing the Republic: The Language of Health and the Culture of Nationalism in Nineteenth-Century America.* New York: Cambridge University Press, 1994.

Burnett, Mary McClellan. "Women Contribute Greatly to Medicine: Andrew Taylor Still Memorial Address." *The DO* 40, no, 10 (Oct. 1999): 55–59.

Burns, Louisa. "Woman's Osteopathic Club Builds House for the A. T. Still Research Institute." *The Western Osteopath* (May 1925): 16.

Bynum, W. F., et al. *The Western Medical Tradition.* New York: Cambridge University Press, 2006.

"California Reopens to DOs." *The DO* 14 (May 1974): 81.

Carpenter, George. "More Women Needed." Letters to the AOA. *Forum of Osteopathy* (April 1953): 5.

Carson, M. J. Open letter. *Journal of Osteopathy* 26, no. 12 (Dec. 1919): 760.

"Change of Editors." *Journal of Osteopathy* 21 (Aug. 1914): 499.

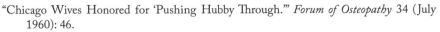

"Chicago Wives Honored for 'Pushing Hubby Through.'" *Forum of Osteopathy* 34 (July 1960): 46.

"The Chronology of Capitulation." *The DO* 1 (Sept. 1961): 35.

"COA Charter Revoked." *AOA News Bulletin* 3 (Nov. 1960): 1.

College of Osteopathic Physicians and Surgeons. *Western Alumnus of the College of Osteopathic Physicians and Surgeons.* N.p.: 1970.

"College Recommended for Federal Grant." *Journal of Osteopathy* 54 (Jan. 1947): 21–22.

Conger, Emily Bronson. *An Ohio Woman in the Philippines: Giving Personal Experiences and Descriptions including Incidents of Honolulu, Ports of Japan and China.* Akron, OH: Press of R. H. Leighton, 1904.

"Constitution of the American Osteopathic Association." *JAOA* 1 (1901): 16–17.

Crosby, Alfred. *Epidemic and Peace, 1918.* Westport, CT: Greenwood Press, 1976.

Crumpler, Rebecca, M.D. *A Book of Medical Discourses in Two Parts...* Boston: Cashman, Keating, 1883.

"Current News: D. O. Heads M-G-M Emergency Hospital." *Forum of Osteopathy* 13 (Sept. 1939): 131–32.

"Death of Jeanette Hubbard Bolles." *Forum of Osteopathy* 4 (April 1930): 14.

"Deaths." *Forum of Osteopathy* 27 (Nov. 1952): 261.

"Des Moines Funds New College." *Osteopathic Physician* 8, no. 1 (June 1905): 1.

DiGiovanna, Eileen L. *An Encyclopedia of Osteopathy.* Indianapolis, IN: American Academy of Osteopathy, 2001.

———, and Stanley Schiowitz. *An Osteopathic Approach to Diagnosis and Treatment.* Philadelphia: Lippincott Williams and Wilkins, 1991.

———, Stanley Schiowitz, and Dennis J. Dowling. *An Osteopathic Approach to Diagnosis and Treatment*, 3rd ed. Philadelphia: Lippincott Williams and Wilkins, 2005.

"Dr. and Mrs. Starks." *The DO* 14 (Feb. 1974): 56–57.

"Dr. Blanche Still Laughlin Dies." *Journal of Osteopathy* 66 (Dec. 1959): 48.

"Dr. Drennan Teaching Plaster Work." *Journal of Osteopathy* 26 (May 1919): 252.

Drexel University School of Medicine. "History, 1848–2002." Accessed 17 Feb. 2011. www.drexelmed.edu/Home/AboutTheCollege/History.aspx.

Duffy, John. *The Healers: A History of American Medicine.* Urbana: University of Illinois Press, 1979.

"Editorials." *Journal of Osteopathy* 21 (May 1914): 302.

"Entrance Requirements, Next Steps." *JAOA* 39 (1939): 225–26.

"The First Woman Doctor of Osteopathy." *Forum of Osteopathy* 4 (April 1930): 14.

Fitzgerald, Mike. "Women in History, Pioneers of the Profession." *The DO* 25 (Dec. 1984): 67–71.

Flexner, Abraham. *Medical Education in the United States and Canada: A Report to the Carnegie Foundation for the Advancement of Teaching.* New York: Carnegie Foundation for the Advancement of Teaching, 1910. Available online at http://www.carnegiefoundation.org/publications/pub.asp?key=43&subkey=977. [Cited as *Flexner Report.*]

Fox, Penny. "Emily Bronson Conger, 1843–1917." *Akron Women's History.* Accessed 8 Nov. 2005. www.uakron.edu/schlcomm/womenshistory/conger_e.htm.

"From President Willard: Materia Medica." *JAOA* 25 (Dec. 1925): 279–80.

"Garson Was a Goner." *Forum of Osteopathy* 13 (Aug. 1939): 98.

Gevitz, Norman. *The DOs: Osteopathic Medicine in America.* 2nd ed. Baltimore: John Hopkins University Press, 2004.

Gevitz, Norman. "The Sword and the Scalpel: The Osteopathic 'War' to Enter the Military Medical Corps: 1916–1966." *JAOA* 98 (May 1998): 279–86.

Grace, Fran. *Carry A. Nation: Retelling the Life.* Bloomington: Indiana University Press, 2001.

"Grace Noll Crowell: Songs out of Suffering." In William L. Stidger, *The Human Side of Greatness,* 3rd ed., 176–94. New York: Harper and Brothers, 1940.

Greenfield, Barbara. "Women Wielding Influence." *The DO* 45 (Dec. 2004): 29.

Gregory, Alva A. *Spinal Treatment.* Oklahoma City: Gregory, 1910. 2nd ed. Oklahoma City: Palmer-Gregory College of Chiropractic, 1912. Citations are to the 2nd edition.

Grigg, E. R. N. "Peripatetic Pioneer: William Smith, MD, DO (1862–1912)." *Journal of the History of Medicine* 22 (April 1967): 169–79.

Gross, Olga. "For Men Only? Active Scope for Practice Offered to Women in the Care of School Athletes." *Osteopathic Profession* 1 (Nov. 1933): 33.

Hacker, Carlotta. *The Indomitable Lady Doctors.* Toronto: Clarke, Irwin, 1974.

Hanaford, Phebe Ann. *Daughters of America; or, Women of the Century.* Augusta, ME: True and Co., [1882].

Hawkins, Peter, and Arthur O'Neill. *Osteopathy in Australia.* Bundoora, Australia: Phillip Institute of Technology, 1990.

Heath, Deborah, and Norman Gevitz. "The Research Status of Somatic Dysfunction." In Ward, *Foundations of Osteopathic Medicine,* 1188–93.

Heffel, Leonard E. *Opportunities in Osteopathic Medicine Today.* Louisville, KY: Vocational Guidance Manuals, 1974.

Heins, Marilyn, Sue Smock, Lois Martindale, Jennifer Jacobs, and Margaret Stein. "Special Communication: Comparison of the Productivity of Women and Men Physicians." *JAMA* 237 (June 1977): 2514–17.

Hildreth, Arthur G. *The Lengthening Shadow of Dr. Andrew Taylor Still.* Kirksville, MO: Journal Printing Company, 1938.

Hodge, L., et al. "JAOA's 50th Annual Research Conference—Abstracts, 2006: Lymphatic Pump Treatment Increases Leukocyte Numbers in Thoracic Duct Lymph." *JAOA* 106 (Aug. 2006): 496.

Holmes, Oliver Wendell. *Medical Essays, 1842–1882.* Boston: Houghton Mifflin, 1892.

Hulett, C. M. Turner. "Historical Sketch of the AAAO." *JAOA* 1 (1900): 1–6.

Hunt, Harriot K. *Glances and Glimpses; or Fifty Years Social, including Twenty Years Professional Life.* Boston: John P. Jewett, 1852.

"Imaginative Vision and Organizational Capacity." *JAOA* 56 (May 1957): 549–50.

"Important Change in Hospital Construction Act Regulations." *JAOA* 46 (1947): 570.

"Infirmary and School Notes." *Journal of Osteopathy* 3 (July 1896): 4.

"In the Mailbag: Royalty's Neck." *Forum of Osteopathy* 14 (June 1940): 50.

Jackson, Robert B. "Andrew Taylor Still, MD, DO, The Man, The Pioneer, The Educator and Founder of Osteopathy." *Chiropractic History* 20, no. 2 (Dec. 2000): 25–26.

James, Laura. *The Love Pirate and the Bandit's Son: Murder, Sin, and Scandal in the Shadow of Jesse James.* New York: Union Square Books, 2009.

Jones, Bob E. *The Difference a D.O. Makes: Osteopathic Medicine in the Twentieth Century.* Oklahoma City, OK: Times-Journal Publishing Co., 1978.

Kett, Joseph F. *The Formation of the American Medical Profession: The Role of Institutions, 1780–1860.* New Haven, CT: Yale University Press, 1968.

King, Hollis. *The Collected Papers of Viola M. Frymann, DO: Legacy of Osteopathy to Children.* Indianapolis, IN: American Academy of Osteopathy, 1998.

Kirschmann, Ann Taylor. *A Vital Force: Women in American Homeopathy.* New Brunswick, NJ: Rutgers University Press, 2004.

Kisch, Arnold I., and Arthur J. Viseltear. *Doctors of Medicine and Doctors of Osteopathy in California: Two Medical Professions Face the Problem of Providing Medical Care.* Arlington, VA: US Dept. of Health, Education and Welfare, Public Health Service, Division of Medical Care Administration, 1967.

Klofkorn, Warren K., and J. Lynne Dodson. *One Hundred Years of Osteopathic Medicine: A Photographic History.* Greenwich, CT: Greenwich Press, 1995.

Korr, Irvin M., et al. *The Physiological Basis of Osteopathic Medicine.* Adapted from the Symposium presented on October 7, 1967. New York: Postgraduate Institute of Osteopathic Medicine and Surgery, 1968.

Leahy, Jack. "How DOs Feel about AOA-AMA Relations." *Osteopathic Physician* 38 (July 1972): 28.

Licciardone, J. C., and K. M. Herron. "Characteristics, Satisfaction, and Perceptions of Patients Receiving Ambulatory Healthcare from Osteopathic Physicians: A Comparative National Survey." *JAOA* 101, no. 7 (July 2001): 374–85.

"Located in Kirksville, Missouri." *Journal of Osteopathy* 2 (Feb. 1896): 8.

"Locations and Removals." *Journal of Osteopathy* 17 (Dec. 1910): 1250.

March, David D., ed. *A Book of Adair County History.* N.p., MO: Simpson Printing Company, 1976.

Mason, J. Louise. "An Osteopath in Turkey." *Journal of Osteopathy* 28 (April 1921): 232 35.
——— ———. "Osteopathy Cures Patients in Turkey." *JAOA* 19 (March 1920): 242.

Mayba, I. I. *Bonesetters and Others: Pioneer Orthopaedic Surgeons.* Winnipeg, Man.: Henderson Books, 1991.

McCole, George. "Osteopathic Definitions." *Forum of Osteopathy* 10 (1936): 151–68.

McNeff, Mary. "The Women's Challenge." *Forum of Osteopathy* 2 (Nov. 1928): 8.

McNiven, Margaret. "Women in Medicine." *Michigan Medicine* (Sept. 1991): 34.

"MDs Can Teach DOs—If." *AOA News Bulletin* 3 (June 1959): 1–2.

"Medical Licensure Statistics for 1970," *JAMA* 216 (14 June 1971): 1786.

"Medical Missionary Returns from Africa." *Journal of Osteopathy* 61 (Sept. 1954): 30.

"Michigan to Establish Osteopathic School," *AOA News Review* 12 (Aug. 1969): 1–2.

Miller, Carol. *A Second Voice: A Century of Osteopathic Medicine in Ohio.* Athens: Ohio University Press, 2004.

Mills, Lawrence W. "Applications to Osteopathic Colleges." *JAOA* 51 (1952): 541–42.
———. "Doctors Wanted: Women Urged to Apply." *Forum of Osteopathy* 20 (Dec. 1946): 289–97.

"A Modern Wonder." *Journal of Osteopathy* 2 (Sept 1895): 7.

Morantz-Sanchez, Regina Markell. *Sympathy and Science: Women Physicians in American Medicine.* New York: Oxford University Press, 1985.

"Mrs. Nettie H. Bolles: Editor and Publisher." *Journal of Osteopathy* 1 (July 1894): 2–3.

Nation, Carrie Amelia. *The Use and Need of the Life of Carrie A. Nation, Written by Herself.* Rev. ed. Topeka, KS: F. M. Steves & Sons, 1908.

"Nature of Osteopathy." *JAMA* 89 (Oct. 1927): 1354–55.

"News of the Month." *Journal of Osteopathy* 25, no. 2 (Feb. 1918): 101.

"A Noble Life-Work." *Journal of Osteopathy* 3 (Nov. 1896): 3.

O'Donnell, Bernard, "The Vampire of Kansas City." In *Kiss and Kill*, edited by Sebastian Wolfe, 215–26. New York: Carroll & Graf Publishers, 1990.

Offen, Karen M. *European Feminisms, 1700–1950: A Political History.* Stanford, CA: Stanford University Press, 2000.

"Official Website of the British Monarchy, The Princess Royal." Accessed 5 Jan. 2011. www. royal.gov.uk/ThecurrentRoyalFamily/ThePrincessRoyal/ThePrincessRoyal.aspx.

Osborne, Robert. *A History of the Oklahoma State University College of Osteopathic Medicine.* Stillwater: Oklahoma State University, 1998.

Osteopathic Center for Children. "Helping all children reach their potential since 1982." Accessed 15 Oct. 2006. www.osteopathiccenter.org/bios.html.

Osteopathic Research Center. "Mission and Goals," updated 5 April 2010. www.hsc.unt. edu/orc.

———. *ORC Annual Report, 2008–2009.* University of North Texas Health Science Center, 2009. Available online at www.hsc.unt.edu/orc/news.html.

"Osteopathic Unit Makes Excellent Showing in Annual Report." *Western Osteopath* 24 (Sept. 1929): 7–10.

"Osteopathic vs. Medical Hospital Efficiency." *JAOA* 32 (1932): 133–35.

"Osteopathy's Epidemic Record." *Osteopathic Physician* 36 (July 1919): 1.

"Osteopathy: Special Report of the Judicial Council to the AMA House of Delegates." *JAMA* 177 (1961): 775.

"Outstanding Woman Doctors: They Make Their Mark in Medicine." *Ebony,* May 1964, 68–76.

Oxford Dictionary of National Biography. Oxford/New York: Oxford University Press, 2004.

Palmer, Daniel David. *The Chiropractor.* 1914. Reprint, N.p.: Kessinger Publishing, 1996.

Parker, Gail Underwood. *Historical Memoirs: The Osteopathic Hospital of Maine Brighton Medical Center, 1935–1998.* Saco, ME: Custom Communications, 2000.

Patterson, Alice. "Why Not Call Our Women Doctors?" *Journal of Osteopathy* 12 (Dec. 1907): 18.

Patterson, Mrs. H. E. (Alice). "Women in Osteopathy." *Journal of Osteopathy* 4 (June 1897): 71–72.

PCOM 1999 Alumni Directory, Centennial Edition. White Plains, NY: Bernard C. Harris Publishing, 1999.

"A Period of Uncertainty." In Pennsylvania Osteopathic Medical Association, *Pennsylvania Osteopathic Medical Association: Supporting Osteopathic Medicine in Pennsylvania for 100 Years.* Harrisburg, PA: Pennsylvania Osteopathic Medical Association, 2003.

"Pennsylvania DO's Back AOA Policies." *Journal of the POMA* 5 (Summer 1963): 8.

Perloff, Carol Benenson. *To Secure Merit: A Century of Philadelphia College of Osteopathic Medicine, 1899–1999.* Philadelphia: Philadelphia College of Osteopathic Medicine, 1999.

"Perseverence Rewarded." *Journal of Osteopathy* 5, no. 6 (Nov. 1898): 273–74.

Potee, Ruth, Andrew Gerber, and Jeannette Ickovics. "Medicine and Motherhood: Shifting Trends among Female Physicians from 1922 to 1999." *Academic Medicine* 74 (Aug. 1999): 911–19.

"A Practical Text-Book on 'Osteopathic Mechanics' Has at Last Been Produced!!!" *The Osteopathic Physician* 30 (Feb. 1916): 1.

"Preserving Heritage, A Retrospective Journey: Tracing the Origins and Development of the Still National Osteopathic Museum." *Now & Then* [SNOM Newsletter] (Spring 2005): 1–17.

"Proceedings of the Fifth Annual Meeting of the AAAO." *JAOA* 1 (1901): 6–15.

"Proceedings of the House of Delegates." *Forum of Osteopathy* 3 (Aug. 1929): supp. 5–8.

"Proceedings of the House of Delegates." *JAOA* 40 (1940): 33–34.

"Program at the Missouri Osteopathic Association." *Journal of Osteopathy* 13 (June 1906): 301.

Quinn, Thomas, and Joseph Byrne. "Physician." In *Encyclopedia of Pestilence, Pandemics, and Plagues*, edited by Joseph Burne, 475–79. Westport, CT: Greenwood, 2008.

Quireshi, Y., and A. Kusienski. "Commentary on the Globalization of Osteopathic Medicine." *Osteopathic Family Physician* 2 (May/June 2010): 72–76.

Reed, C.C. "Prevention and Treatment of Influenza." *JAOA* 18, no. 1 (1919): 209–11.

"Red Cross Authorized DOs." *Forum of Osteopathy* 26 (Oct. 1952): 201–2.

"Report of the Committee for the Study of Relations between Osteopathy and Medicine." *JAMA* 158 (2 July 1955): 736–42.

"Report of the Judicial Council." *JAMA* 171, no. 7 (17 Oct. 1959): 978–79.

Riley, George W. "Osteopathy's First Half Century." *JAOA* 23 (July 1924): 821–22.

Riley, George. "Osteopathy's Power over Flu-Pneumonia." *Osteopathic Physician* 36 (July 1919): 6.

Riley, George W. "Professional Duty and Opportunity." *JAOA* 17 (Aug. 1918): 654–62.

Rogers, John. "Report of the Bureau of Professional Education and Colleges." *JAOA* 36 (1937): 607.

Rosenblatt, Roger A., et al, "Which Medical Schools Produce Rural Physicians?" *JAMA* 268 (23/30 Sept. 1992): 1559–65.

Rossiter, Margaret W. *Women Scientists in America: Struggles and Strategies to 1940.* Baltimore: Johns Hopkins University Press, 1982.

Schiebinger, Londa. *The Mind Has No Sex? Women in the Origins of Science.* Cambridge, MA: Harvard University Press, 1989.

"The Science of Osteopathy." *The Osteopath* 1 (Feb. 1897): 4.

Sexton, Christine. "Working 9 to 3." *Florida Medical Business* 22 (May 2008): 1–12.

Simpson, M. A., and M. A. Weiser. "Studying the Impact of Women on Osteopathic Physician Workforce Predictions." *JAOA* 96 (Feb. 1996): 106–11.

Smith, Georgia. "What the OWNA Is Doing for Osteopathy." *Clinical Osteopathy* (April 1940): 226–29.

Smith, Wm. "Reviews Pioneer Days." *Osteopathic Physician* 3 (Jan. 1903): 1.

Smith, Wm. "Four Years Ago, Dr. Wm. Smith Gives an Account of His First Visit to Dr. Still." *Journal of Osteopathy* 3 (Sept. 1896): 6.

"Some Foolish Things to Be Dropped." *Journal of Osteopathy* 10, no. 4 (April 1903): 8.

Spraycar, Marjory, ed. *Stedman's Medical Dictionary.* 26th ed. Baltimore, MD: Williams and Williams, 1995.

Srofe, Bessie. "Osteopath in Salvation Army over There." *Journal of Osteopathy* 26 (March 1919): 145–48.

Starr, Paul. *The Social Transformation of American Medicine.* New York: Basic Books, 1982.

Still, Andrew T. *Autobiography of Andrew Taylor Still.* Kirksville, MO, 1897.

———. "Dr. Still's Department." *Journal of Osteopathy* 6, no. 3 (Aug. 1899).

———. *Osteopathy Research and Practice.* Kirksville, MO: The author, 1910.

———. "Our Platform." *Journal of Osteopathy* 9, no, 10 (Oct. 1902): 342.

———. "Recollections of Baldwin, Kansas." *Journal of Osteopathy* 1, no. 9 (Jan. 1895): 2.

Still, Blanche. "A Soldier's Story from the Spanish American War." *Journal of Osteopathy* 5, no. 5 (Oct. 1898): 246-47.

Still, Charles E., Jr. *Frontier Doctor, Medical Pioneer: The Life and Times of A. T. Still and His Family.* Kirksville, MO: Thomas Jefferson University Press at Northeast Missouri State University, 1991.

"Sullivan and Maugham." *Journal of Osteopathy* 46 (Feb. 1939); 8.

"Supplemental Report of the Board of Trustees." *JAMA* 156 (1954): 1600–1605.

"TCOM Becomes State-Supported Medical School as Governor Briscoe Signs SB 216." *Texas Osteopathic Physician Journal* 32 (July 1975): 12–13.

"Text of Michigan Resolution." *AOA News Bulletin* 3 (Aug. 1959): 1–3.

Thiessen, Carol. "Greenbriar: The Little College that Could." *The DO* 15 (March 1975): 82–92.

Tilley, R. McFarlane. "Osteopathic Education." *Forum of Osteopathy* 25 (April 1951): 23.

"To Inspect the Mayo Hospital," *Journal of Osteopathy* 15 (October 1908): 638.

Trowbridge, Carol. *Andrew Taylor Still, 1828–1917.* Kirksville, MO: Truman State University Press, 1991.

Tucker, E.E. "Spanish Influenza: What and Why." *JAOA* 18, no. 6 (Feb. 1919): 270–73.

University of Bedfordshire. "Princess Royal Presents Degrees to First Osteopathy Graduates," 24 November 2005. Accessed 17 March 2007. www.beds.ac.uk/news/2005/nov/051124-bso.

University of Bedfordshire. "Royal Seal of Approval for Uni Graduates," 11 November 2010. Accessed 5 Jan. 2011. www.beds.ac.uk/news/2010/nov/101111-bso.

Urban and Rural Systems Associates. *Women in Osteopathic Medicine.* Vol. 3 of *Exploratory Study of Women in the Health Professions Schools.* Washington, DC: US Dept. of Health, Education, and Welfare, Women's Action Program, 1976.

"Veteran's Administration." *Journal of Osteopathy* 54, no. 1 (Jan. 1947): 25.

Veazie, D. B. Open Letter. *Journal of Osteopathy* 26, no. 12 (Dec. 1919): 760.

Violette, E. M. *History of Adair County.* Kirksville, MO: Denslow History Co., 1911.

Walsh, Mary Ruth. *Doctors Wanted: No Women Need Apply.* New Haven, CT: Yale University Press, 1977.

Walter, Georgia W. *The First School of Osteopathic Medicine.* Kirksville, MO: Thomas Jefferson University Press at Northeast Missouri State University, 1992.

———. *Women and Osteopathic Medicine.* Kirksville, MO: National Center for Osteopathic History, 1994.

Ward, Robert C., ed. *Foundations for Osteopathic Medicine.* 2nd ed. Philadelphia: Lippincott Williams and Wilkins, 2002.

"Washington State MD-DO Plan Told." *AMA News* 6 (11 November 1963): 16.

"What ERA Means to Osteopaths." *Achievement* 2 (April 1923): 5–10.

Who's Who. "Unusual Honor for Dr. Morelock." *Forum of Osteopathy* 1, no. 5 (Aug. 1927): 22.

Willard, A. "Where Our Students Come From." *JAOA* 46 (1947): 313.

World Osteopathic Helath Organization. Accessed 2 July 2009. www.woho.org.

Wright, Harry. *Perspectives in Osteopathic Medicine.* Kirksville, MO: Kirksville College of Osteopathic Medicine, 1976.

Zornow, William F. *Kansas: A History of the Jayhawk State.* Norman: University of Oklahoma Press, 1957.

ARCHIVES AND ABBREVIATIONS

ACOS	American College of Osteopathic Surgeons
AOA Archives	American Osteopathic Association Archives, Chicago, IL
ASO	American School of Osteopathy, Kirksville, MO
JAOA	*Journal of the American Osteopathic Association*
JAMA	*Journal of the American Medical Association*
MOM	Museum of Osteopathic Medicine (sm), Kirksville, MO
NCOH	National Center for Osteopathic History, Kirksville, MO
PCO	Philadelphia College of Osteopathy
PCOM	Philadelphia College of Osteopathic Medicine
POMA	Pennsylvania Osteopathic Medical Association

YEARBOOKS

Cortex	Yearbook of College of Osteopathic Physicians and Surgeons, Los Angeles
The Nucleolus	Yearbook of Los Angeles College of Osteopathy
Osteoblast	Yearbook of American School of Osteopathy, Kirksville, MO
Synapsis	Yearbook of Philadelphia College of Osteopathy/Philadelphia College of Osteopathic Medicine

About the Author

THOMAS A. QUINN, DO, FAOCOPM, is a graduate of the Philadelphia College of Osteopathic Medicine and is board certified in occupational medicine and family practice. Dr. Quinn was one of the first osteopathic physicians to be commissioned as a medical officer in the US Navy, where he served on active duty for two years. After being discharged, Dr. Quinn was in private practice in Lancaster, Pennsylvania, for twenty-two years while he continued to serve in the Navy Reserve and Pennsylvania Army National Guard. Dr. Quinn has served as commander of the 103rd Medical Battalion, division surgeon of the 28th Infantry Division, and state surgeon of the Pennsylvania National Guard.

Since 1990, Dr. Quinn has practiced occupational medicine and served as the national medical director for Humana Workers' Compensation Services and as the Medical Director for the Florida League of Cities. He joined the faculty of the Lake Erie College of Osteopathic Medicine, Bradenton in 2005, where he continues to teach. Dr. Quinn is married; he has two children and two grandchildren.